New hope, new health...

From the author of *Be Your Own Best Friend* and *Increase Your Energy*, this important guide illustrates just how powerful a role we can play in our health and well-being—with discussions of the nature of illness and the importance of harnessing the mind's potential, as well as easy-to-use alternative tools including...

- affirmations and visualization
- chakra work
- Bach flower remedies
- relaxation techniques
- reflexology

  and more

SELF-HEALING
USE YOUR MIND TO HEAL YOUR BODY

Berkley titles by Louis Proto

SELF-HEALING
INCREASE YOUR ENERGY
BE YOUR OWN BEST FRIEND

SELF-
HEALING

LOUIS PROTO

BERKLEY BOOKS, NEW YORK

To my Mother and Father

SELF-HEALING

A Berkley Book / published by arrangement with
Samuel Weiser, Inc.

PRINTING HISTORY
Piatkus Publishers Ltd. edition published 1990
Samuel Weiser, Inc. edition published 1991
Berkley edition / November 1997

The Putnam Berkley World Wide Web site address is
http://www.berkley.com

ISBN: 0-425-16192-7

BERKLEY®
Berkley Books are published by The Berkley Publishing Group,
a member of Penguin Putnam Inc.,
200 Madison Avenue, New York, New York 10016.
BERKLEY and the "B" design
are trademarks belonging to Berkley Publishing Corporation.

PRINTED IN THE UNITED STATES OF AMERICA

10 9 8 7 6 5 4 3 2 1

CONTENTS

PART III • WELLNESS

ACKNOWLEDGMENTS

I should like to express thanks to: Pat Pilkington, co-founder of the Bristol Cancer Help Centre, for her encouragement and support, and for allowing me to quote from one of her letters to me; Louise Hay for being a continuing source of inspiration; Caroline Myss for opening up a whole new way of looking at illness—and making me laugh a lot in the process; Martin Brofman for generously allowing the use of his chart of the chakras and teaching me how to heal through them; Gabrielle Pinto for clarifying the finer points of homoeopathy; Isabel Maxwell Cade for the charts showing Alpha and Beta brainwave patterns; the Bach Centre, England, for kindly allowing publication of the Bach Remedies; and to the following publishers for giving permission to quote from their books:

Century Hutchinson (*Love, Medicine and Miracles* by Bernie Siegel and *The Bristol Programme* by Penny Brohn); Gateway Books (*Maximum Immunity* by Michael Weiner); The CW Daniel Company, Ltd. (*Subtle Energy* by John Davidson); Bantam Books, Inc. (*Getting Well Again* by Carl Simonton, Stephanie Matthews-Simonton and James L. Creighton); Arkana (*Self-Healing: My Life and Vision* by Meir Scheider).

ACKNOWLEDGMENTS

PREFACE

Sitting one day in my garden by the pool (not a swimming pool, but a beautiful little fishpond), wrestling with the problems of structuring this book and more than a little dismayed by the sheer volume of my research notes, I chanced across an observation by Simon Martin in the foreword to John Davidson's book *Subtle Energy*. It read:

> It seems that never before have we had access to so much information about the way our bodies and minds work . . . We already have more than enough information to absolutely transform our lifestyles, our health, and the planet who supports us, so that we can achieve the high evolutionary purpose I believe we are here for. *The problem is not a lack of information: the problem is a lack of people who can synthesize vast amounts of information, add it up and then simplify it for mass communication.* (My italics)

Thank you, Simon, for those words that transformed my labour into a labour of love. And appropriately so, for that is what healing yourself ultimately is.

AUTHOR'S NOTE

Affirmations and visualisations are used throughout this book. If you haven't come across these before, you may find it helpful to turn to pages 113–127 after reading the introduction.

It should be stressed that in no way is the information given in this book intended to replace treatment by a registered medical practitioner. Rather, it is a way of sharing with you the experiences of other people who are ill, often very seriously, and who are managing successfully to find relief—and in many cases remission or cure—from their ailments. They have achieved this through self-healing in conjunction with medical care. Your doctor should be kept informed of how you are trying to assist in your own healing process, to enhance the effectiveness of any treatment he may give you and to minimise side effects. If in any doubt, ask for his or her advice.

FOREWORD

by Louise L. Hay

When Dan Olmos, one of my editors, first came to me with a proposal to write a foreword for *Self-Healing*, I must confess that I was not overly enthusiastic. Due to my lecture commitments and my own writing projects, as well as the everyday processes of running a publishing company, I find it difficult to find time to *read* a book, let alone write a foreword for one I know nothing about.

However, Dan didn't ask for my decision right then. He, perhaps too wisely, left the manuscript on my desk where he knew I would get to it quickly due to my preference for an uncluttered desk.

Later, that same afternoon, I started leafing through the manuscript—quickly at first, then slower . . . and slower, until I found myself reading it word for word. Louis Proto has written a wonderfully informative book for anyone interested in the principles of self-healing. He has taken the guesswork out of searching for alternative methods of healing and lumped them together in one magnificent book! And now, here I am writing the foreword.

I have often said that I am a simple lady with a simple message: Love your self, heal your life. When someone comes to me with a problem, regardless of what it is, there is only one thing I ever suggest that he or she work on, and that is *loving the self*. I find that when we really love, accept and approve of our selves exactly as we are, then everything else in life ticks and tocks along like clockwork. We see the light, so to speak, and little miracles begin to appear everywhere.

But what happens if we don't "see the light" until it's too late? Until our physical body is very sick? What changes can we possibly make then?

First of all, I believe it is never too late to begin to love your self more, just as it is never too early. Loving your self also means listening to what your body is telling you. When your body is sick, it is telling you that something is wrong; there is something you have neglected and it is up to you to find out what it is and to do what is necessary to nourish your self back to health.

When I was first diagnosed with cancer of the vagina, I did what everyone else in that situation does—I panicked. And that was after I had already written a book, was counselling clients and speaking on the lecture circuit!

After I calmed myself down, I was able to see my cancer as an opportunity to prove to myself that self-healing works. I had written *Heal Your Body* and I knew that cancer was a dis-ease caused by deep resentment that had been held for a long time until it literally ate away at the body. I also knew that my resentment came from my past of physical and sexual abuse. That meant I had a lot of work to do.

I convinced my doctor to give me some time and I set out on a most important journey—a journey within my self. I went to several health food stores and bought every book they had on cancer. I went to the local library and checked out even more. I read as much as I could on the subject, then went about exploring the therapies that I felt would benefit me the most. I worked with a foot reflexologist, a nutritionist and a colonic therapist. I found a good personal therapist who helped me express my anger by beating on pillows and screaming with rage.

As my inner self grew, so did my understanding of the resentments I had held on to for so long. Blame slowly melted into compassion and my cancer melted with it. In six months my doctor confirmed what I already knew. I no longer had cancer.

I had chosen the course of action that was right for me.

Today, people come to me and ask me to provide a therapy that will work for their particular health situation.

I can make suggestions and I can definitely explain what worked for me, but ultimately each individual has to take full responsibility for their selves and know that the course they have chosen is the best one for them.

Meditation is a wonderful way to connect with your inner self and get answers to the questions you seek. If we would only take the time to listen to our inner selves more often, there is no telling how many problems we could overcome on our own.

In *Self-Healing*, Louis Proto provides readers with the tools they need to make their own inner journeys. Meditation, visualisation, detoxification, vitamin supplements, massage, reflexology, acupuncture, accupressure, Bach flower remedies, affirmations, chakra work and my favourite, of course, loving the self, are all dutifully represented in his text. Let yourself read about the different therapies available and investigate the ones that seem right for you. You will know which ones they are. Just listen to that little voice inside your head and go with what it tells you. Explore, explore, and explore some more!

Remember, there is never one right way to do anything. I have often head that "there are many spokes to the centre of the wheel." I feel that way about our health. We are each unique, divine expressions of life and we all have our own unique, divine way of handling our health situations. Some may choose, like I did, to do healing work all by themselves. Others may choose to rely solely on the wonders of modern medicine. And others may choose a happy medium and combine the two.

I personally never tell people to abandon their doctors. Many are not ready to do that. Instead I tell them to work in conjunction with their doctors and get the best of both worlds. But most important, I emphasise that they must participate in and feel good about the treatment they are receiving. They must trust their Higher Power that it is the right treatment for them.

In chapter four of this book, Louis Proto writes, "Choosing to accept a share in responsibility for creating sickness in our bodies is in fact to move out of the position of victim, and to take back the power to heal ourselves. *For what we can create, we can choose to stop creating.*'' Emphasis mine. Mr. Proto is making a very important point and one that is worth repeating—*What you create, you can uncreate.* I firmly believe this.

The more power you accept in yourself, the more confident you will become of your individual abilities. And with that confidence will grow your self-esteem and self-love. When you feel good about yourself, you feel good, period.

Use *Self-Healing* as a catalyst in exploring the health options that are available for you. Take responsibility for your health. Learn to trust your health. And above all, *love your health*, whatever it may be. Then, watch the wonderfully miraculous things that will happen for you . . . and rejoice.

Louise L. Hay
Hay House
November 1989

INTRODUCTION

There is no such thing as an incurable illness. Anything can be healed. That this is so is shown by the example of individuals who had the courage to accept a dire diagnosis as a challenge instead of a death sentence, a passionate desire to go on living, a willingness to change the patterns that had laid them low, the determination to participate in their own healing and the knowledge of how to do so, and enough vital force left in their bodies to enable them to make a 180 degree turn in the direction of a restoration to health.

Here are a few such examples of survivors from catastrophic illness. They are alive and well today and helping others to heal themselves.

Louise Hay

Louise Hay had cancer of the vagina. Received news of the diagnosis "with total panic"—then got down to changing her diet, letting go of the long-standing resentment to do with her abuse as a child, and using the power of the mind to heal the body. Total cure within six months. Now, as a "metaphysical teacher" practising in California, and through her books and tapes, is teaching many others that "dissolving patterns dissolves disease."

Martin Brofman

Former Wall Street executive. Diagnosed with throat cancer in 1975 and given only months to live. Healed himself by learning how to work with energy at subtle levels. Now an internationally known healer conducting healing intensives worldwide.

Penny Brohn

Tells the story in *Gentle Giants* (see Further Reading) of how, in 1979, disillusioned with conventional treatment, she "fled from England with a bruised, leaky wound in my breast, a bag of sterile dressings and the terrifying diagnosis of a carcinoma" to the Dr. Josef Issels Ringbergklinik. Co-founder with Pat Pilkington of the Bristol Cancer Help Centre which has pioneered the "gentle way with cancer" using the holistic approaches she describes in *The Bristol Programme* (see Further Reading).

Katherina Collins

One of the Bristol Centre's many "successes." A classic example of the link between loss and catastrophic illness, she was diagnosed with breast cancer soon after her husband died following a six year illness through which she had nursed him. She restored herself to health by totally transforming her diet, mental attitudes, and ways of relating. One of the things she had to give up was being compulsively "nice," and one of the things she had to learn was how to accept love. Katherina is still in remission and keeps herself busy with her London support group which now numbers 600. They are raising funds for a house in East London to turn into a full Cancer Help Centre.

Norman Cousins

Diagnosed in 1964 with ankylosing spondylitis, a painful, crippling and untreatable disease. He describes in his best-seller

Anatomy of an Illness (see Further Reading) how he cured himself—with laughter and high doses of vitamin C. It was when he decided that his massive prescribed doses of pain-killers (26 aspirin tablets and 12 phenylbutazone a day) were doing him no good and he sent out for *Candid Camera* videos and old Marx Brothers films that he started on the road to recovery from what he had been told was an incurable disease.

William Calderon

The first documented recovery from AIDS. Diagnosed in 1982, he was given six months to live. He developed Kaposi's sarcoma, an aggresive form of skin cancer, a common result of the collapse of the body's immune system. After a period of total depression and hopelessness he learned of the work of the Simontons in healing cancer patients using mental imagery. He began trying this for himself, practising meditation and achieving peace of mind through improving his relationship with his family and forgiving those who had ever hurt him. He also cared more for his body with good nutrition, food supplements and exercise. His immune system started to show improved response and his KS lesions began to disappear. Within two years of the initial diagnosis Calderon showed no signs of AIDS.

Louis Nassaney

Louis Nassaney was diagnosed with Kaposi's sarcoma in May 1983. After seven months of identifying with the role of "AIDS victim" he began, with the support of his father and guidance of Louise Hay, to participate in his own healing using vitamin therapy, exercise, acupuncture, visualisation, affirmations, deep relaxation and meditation. After four months, his lesions began to fade and in October 1984 a biopsy revealed only dead scar tissue. He has been described as being "in complete remission" and has been touring the USA bringing messages of hope to other AIDS "victims."

Meir Schneider

Born blind. Underwent five unsuccessful eye operations and was declared incurably (and legally) blind at the age of seven. Ten years later, determined to see, he began to use exercises, breathing techniques and mental imagery to attempt to heal himself. He now reads without glasses and works as a healer. He founded the Centre for Conscious Vision in San Francisco in 1977 and the Centre for Self-Healing in 1980. His work is based on the empowerment of the individual and the stimulation of the natural healing powers of the body. In his book *Self-Healing, My Life and Vision* (see Further Reading) he gives detailed case-histories of some remarkable improvements that have occurred in "incurable diseases." Here are a few.

Rachel

A 40-year-old woman stricken with osteoarthritis which had affected her whole body for a year but was now concentrated in one knee. The knee had swollen to more than twice the size of the other. Within a few months of changing her diet, using deep breathing, massage and visualisation, the pain and swelling in her knee had lessened. Within six months, her arthritis was imperceptible.

Lili

Now five years old, Lili had shown the first symptoms of muscular dystrophy at eighteen months and could barely crawl. She was very weak and thin, and any normal motion was almost impossible for her, including lifting her arms or legs. Massage and remedial exercises strengthened Lili's muscles so effectively that after seven sessions she was able to crawl on hands and knees and, a few weeks later with some support, took her first steps in three years. Soon she was able (once again with some support) to walk down the stairs. Meir Schneider comments:

"This was the most rapid, dramatic progress I have ever

seen with a muscular dystrophy patient. The joy of seeing this little girl on her feet was so powerful it has never left me. She was one of our most astonishing cases. It took only 21 days for her transformation from near-paralysis to walking.''

Stephen

Caroline Myss's first success story as a clairvoyant diagnostician. Stephen followed her intuitive advice of what he needed to do to heal himself of AIDS. He achieved this in six weeks— not just remission, there was not a trace of the virus left in his body. Since Stephen, Caroline has had three more total cures from AIDS.

George Melton and Will Garcia

In his book *Beyond Aids* (see Further Reading), George Melton describes the journey of healing and self-discovery made by himself and his partner Will after they were diagnosed with AIDS in 1985. They refused to accept death as inevitable and, despite the climate of general doom and hysteria, were determined to discover the means by which to live. Within a year they had dispensed completely with drugs and have remained symptom free ever since. They are now helping others to follow their example.

HOPE FOR THE FUTURE

Without doubt there are very many more people successfully healing themselves than we ever hear about. The stories of those who have ''gone public'' are an inspiration to those who find themselves in similar situations and a useful corrective to the gloom and paranoia regularly dished out by the media, particularly about AIDS. For, as we shall be seeing, one of the most powerful agents of healing is *belief*. And if you do not believe that it is possible for you to be healed, then it is very possible that you won't be. Prognoses of having only a few months to live, or being told that something is "invariably fatal" are in fact death sentences; such is the nature of our minds that these pronouncements become self-fulfilling prophecies.

But the implications are wider. After all, if you can heal AIDS and cancer, you can heal anything. And if you are fortunate enough to be already enjoying good health, reading about how others have healed themselves will teach you what works and what doesn't (and maybe explain the reasons why you are staying healthy). You will have a blueprint for staying well and keeping out of trouble in the future. From the holistic point of view, the essential difference between cancer or AIDS, for example, and the common cold is that with cancer and AIDS one is sick at a much deeper level—and therefore one has to work for healing at a much deeper level.

What do we mean by holistic? We mean seeing the person as a *whole* and not just as a body with symptoms to be got rid of. It means seeing the presence of health or the absence of it in terms of energy—whether there is enough of it, whether it is balanced and flowing, or whether it is blocked and stagnating. Healing (as opposed to the mere eradication of symptoms which have manifested in the body as a result of energy imbalance and blockage) is the restoration of harmony at all levels—mental, physical, emotional and spiritual. And the type of healing described in this book—that works with *energy*—is nonspecific: it doesn't matter what the disease is. Change the energy pattern and you change the disease which is its manifestation.

From a homoeopathic point of view, the use of drastic methods to get rid of symptoms (which are the body's distress signals) is to kill the messenger who brings bad news. Sometimes, in acute or life-threatening conditions, resorting to antibiotics or surgery may be essential just to stay alive. But more is needed if disease is not to be driven deeper into our systems, to surface somewhere else at a later date, and perhaps in more virulent form. If the disease has gone so deep already that it is beyond the reach of drugs or surgery, it has become what we mean when we say it is "incurable."

This book will tell you how to participate in your own healing process if you are ill and how to stay well if you are not.

It is in no way intended to supplant conventional medical treatment. Rather, it is an attempt to share how others have supplemented such conventional treatments with self-healing techniques that render the treatments more effective, minimise side effects, and make the patient feel a whole lot better in the process. Here, as always, it is a question of balance, and we have to find our own. Your doctor should be kept informed of how you are trying to help yourself get well and his or her advice sought if at any time you have any doubts or queries. It is probably true to say that most doctors today are coming to see the value of good nutrition, relaxation, positive attitudes and reducing stress, and are beginning to recognise the psychosomatic factors behind all illness. Some, too, are trained in acupuncture or homoeopathy.

See this book, therefore, as a compendium of self-healing techniques that have been proven to work for many people. Use it to find the techniques which will work best for you—to heal yourself of illness or to maintain and improve your health. Choose from the "menus" on offer the ones which will be nourishing for you. Self-healing is an intensely personal affair. Trust your intuition. At some level we always know what we must do to heal ourselves.

part one

ILLNESS

*In the final analysis, we must love
in order not to fall ill.*

—FREUD

one

THE NATURE OF ILLNESS

Louis Pasteur was a truly great man. Not the least part of his greatness was his honesty in admitting he had been wrong. Pasteur's belief that microbes caused disease had been contested by Claude Bernard, who claimed that unless the body's "terrain" was favourable to bacterial invasion, microbes were powerless. In other words, lowered resistance, not germs, was the significant factor in the genesis of disease. At the end of his life, Pasteur murmured to the friends gathered by his deathbed, "Bernard was right, the microbes are nothing. It is the terrain."

It is perhaps not so remarkable that this last insight of one of the world's greatest scientists into the causality of illness should have gone almost unnoticed for the last 80 years or so. In an age such as ours, which has been accustomed to looking outside ourselves for the answers and especially to trusting science to come up with them, there is more comfort in Pasteur than in Bernard. After all, if germs cause disease, it's nothing really to do with us, our lifestyles, our way of being in the world. Disease just "happens," an unfortunate accident for which we have no responsibility. And so, just as we give the power to make us ill over to the infinitely small, so we look up to the towering authority of the medical establishment to make us well again. Ideally with a pill of some sort.

Since Pasteur's death, medical science (backed by the pharmaceutical corporations aware of the fortunes to be made by meeting public demand for "magic bullets") has poured its talent and resources into researching the world of micro-organisms—the bacteria and the viruses—and into developing chemical substances to kill them. And of course many of us who have recovered from acute illnesses with the aid of an-tibiotics have every reason to be grateful for the discovery of these drugs. Overall, our health has improved. More babies survive, and we live longer (though this is probably more due to other factors like a cleaner water supply, better diet and less harsh working conditions, as well as to more effective means of controlling the spread of epidemics).

But there are signs that our trust in the "magic bullet" to heal all our ills is beginning to fade. Before even the advent of the cunning little chameleon that we have labelled HTLV-III, (the AIDS virus capable of transmuting itself to shake off pursuing researchers bent on its destruction) we were begin-ning to get alarmed about the incidence of heart disease and to be curious about why more men succumb to it than women.

Over the last decade, we have become more aware of con-nections between what we put into our bodies, and the stress we put ourselves under, and our state of health. We have been alerted to the dangers of cholesterol, food additives, smoking, lead and other forms of environmental pollution. The inability of our GPs to offer succour (in the absence of identifiable symptoms) to the majority of patients who crowd their sur-geries complaining merely of "feeling unwell" has led many to explore what used to be called "fringe medicine" and has led to a boom in acupuncture, homoeopathy and other "alter-native" therapies. More and more people are seeking relief for their tension and malaise in things other than addiction-producing tranquillisers; for example autogenics, transcenden-tal meditation or jogging.

We are beginning to get the message that maintaining our health is our own responsibility, and that the true role of the professional medic is merely to carry out repairs when things are going wrong.

THE HIT AND MISS NATURE OF DISEASE

Following the germ theory, people develop cholera if they are exposed to the bacterium *vibrio cholerae*, and typhoid if they are exposed to *salmonella typhi*. In 1892, however, this was dramatically shown to be not always the case. The Bavarian scientist Max von Pettenkofer challenged Robert Koch's claim to have discovered the microbe that caused cholera. Pettenkofer secured a sample of the bacillus from a fatal case, poured it into a glass of water and downed it before medical witnesses, with a defiant cry of "Skol!" Far from coming down with the dreaded cholera, all he suffered was a mild case of diarrhoea. His experiment was later repeated by others, with equal success.

Perhaps this spectacular demonstration is not so surprising when we consider that our environment (and our bodies) teem with potentially dangerous organisms all the time. There is simply no way we can avoid continuous exposure to germs short of sealing ourselves up in a totally sterile plastic bubble for the rest of our lives.

Sir Macfarlane Burnet, a Nobel prizewinner for his work on immunology, has stated that within our bodies each day there could be as many as 100,000 cells becoming cancerous—but our immune system destroys them. It has been suggested that we become *infected* (as opposed to producing symptoms) with a cold on average once a month.

The question is not whether bacteria and viruses cause diseases, but why they cause disease in some people and not others? Why do some workers in a busy office go down with the cold or a bug that's "going around," and others don't? Why do some customers of an infected prostitute contract venereal disease while others do not? Why do some HIV-positive individuals go on to develop AIDS when others don't? If mere exposure to germs were enough to cause disease, then the greatest healing shrine in the world would have been closed long ago. Over the years since Bernadette's visions of the Virgin Mary at Lourdes in 1858, millions of pilgrims, many terminally ill and some with open sores and lesions, have bathed in the same spring water at the healing grotto. There has never been a case of anyone being infected.

THE IMMUNE SYSTEM

The advent of AIDS has served to highlight the paramount importance of the body's own defences and self-healing mechanisms in keeping us alive and well. We are now being forced to learn more and more about the nature of these inner defences, how they work, and what strengthens or undermines them. And what a marvellously complex, intelligent and astute system it is.

Under a microscope, a drop of blood taken from a healthy person reveals its content as about 99% of red blood cells and the remaining 1% of white cells (on average, about 5 million red cells and 7,000 white cells per cubic millimetre of blood sampled). These white cells are the "soldiers" of the immune system. Like real soldiers, their job is to be on the look-out for the enemy (invading microbes) and to locate and destroy them. Once again, as in a real army which contains specialised branches in intelligence, signals, artillery and so forth, their contribution to the overall exercise is differentiated according to function. Thus our immune system contains B cells, T cells and macrophages.

Both B and T cells are born in the liver while we are still in the womb. From there they move to the bone marrow. The B cells remain there ("B" stands for "bone marrow-derived") but the T cells migrate to the thymus gland situated in the upper chest ("T" stands for "thymus-derived").

B cells produce antibodies to neutralise, very specifically, each antigen or foreign invader. Antigens could be not only bacteria or viruses, but also dust, fungi, pollen, harmful chemicals—anything, in fact, that triggers off the alarm system.

T cells influence the body's other cells. For example, T helper cells induce the B cells to respond to the antigen, while T suppressor cells (as the name suggests) "switch off" cell activity to avoid overkill when the danger is past. The ratio of T suppressors to T helpers is today seen to indicate the health of the immune system. Normally the ratio is 1.8 helper cells to each suppressor cell (1.8:1). Too many suppressor cells can mean that the immune system is being "switched off," and AIDS patients often reveal a ratio of 1:1 or less.

As well as these B and T cells, our inner defence system

includes large white cells, produced once again in the bone marrow, called macrophages. Once an antigen has been identified, they will simply gobble it up.

Another name for the various components of the immune system is the lymphatic system, and its primary organs are the bone marrow and the thymus. The thymus gland is now recognised as being of key importance in maintaining our immunity to disease. A curious thing about it is that after childhood it begins to shrink and therefore decreases in size relative to body weight. Another significant—and very encouraging—fact for the purposes of this inquiry into self-healing is that the brain can be made to control the functioning of the immune system. We shall be exploring how this can be done in Part II of this book, and learning how to stimulate the thymus and prevent its shrinking further.

It is beyond the scope of this simplified account of the immune system to go into the functions of the secondary organs of immunity: the lymph nodes, spleen, tonsils, appendix, Peyer's patches, and the specialised lymph nodules in the intestinal membranes. By now we will have understood why germs really find it hard to get through our natural defences to make us ill. Unless, that is, we are under too much stress.

Stress and Immunity

That stress depresses immunity is now too well documented to be held in doubt. American scientist Michael Plaut has been researching the effects of stress on the immune systems of mice. He has found that exposing them to a combination of bright lights and repeated electric shocks significantly lowered their production of antibodies. Damaged immunity was also exhibited by mice that had been isolated from their fellows.

In the mid-1970s, Vernon Riley of the Seattle Pacific North West Research Foundation found that in experiments on rats bred to be susceptible to breast cancer, he was able to vary the rate of cancer from 7% to 92% simply by varying their exposure to stress. (In 1956 in his trail-blazing work *The Stress of Life*, Sir Hans Selye, Professor of Experimental Medicine at Montreal's McGill University, had described how the heart muscle of rats put under stress in the laboratory underwent the same acute disintegration that had been found in autopsies on human beings who had died from heart attacks after exposure to stress.)

In February 1986, a four-year study of 2,163 women who reported for breast screening resulted in findings which linked breast cancer statistically to stress. As far back as 1926, Elida Evans, a Jungian analyst who was researching into cancer and its causes, had been struck by the fact that all of her patients who had breast cancer had recently suffered the loss of an important relationship. In 1957, the consulting surgeon at Guy's Hospital in London, Sir Heneage Ogilvie, had startled his colleagues by asserting that "the happy man never gets cancer." His remark echoes that of Sir James Paget, who in the last century stated his view that the real cause of cancer was disappointment.

Of all major life events, the most stressful have been found to be: death of a spouse and divorce or marital separation.

In 1981, researchers at Westminster Hospital discovered that sufferers from rheumatoid arthritis suffered their first attack soon after bereavement, divorce or losing their job. At Mount Sinai in New York, Stephen Scliefer and his colleagues reported that a group of widowers had more depressed immune systems two months after their wives died as compared with immune testing before their bereavement. Separation and divorce have been found to increase mortality from TB and pneumonia in both sexes. At Ohio State University it has also been found that there is more herpes activity in women recently separated or divorced. Apparently, the more these women had loved their husbands, the greater their immune systems had been damaged. The same university reported that there was more herpes activity and less immune reactivity among those students who felt stressed by exams than by those who did not.

Too much stress can cause *anything* from a cold to cancer, from a headache to what used to be called a "nervous breakdown." In 1958, research at McGill University revealed that of 40 sufferers from multiple sclerosis, all but five had been under prolonged stress before their illness manifested itself, and relapse usually followed on the heels of renewed stress.

At the Albert Einstein College of Medicine in the Bronx, it was found that children with cancer had suffered twice as many recent crises as other children, and that 31 out of 33 children with leukemia had experienced a traumatic loss or move within the two years preceding diagnosis.

In 1969, Thomas Holmes and Richard Rahe examined specific events that seemed to precipitate illness in a group of 5,000 patients. They quantified the illness-producing potential of each form of stress as shown in the table below.

The Holmes/Rahe Social Readjustment Rating Scale

Life Event	Score
Death of spouse	100
Divorce	73
Marital separation	65
Prison or mental hospital confinement	63
Death of a close family member	63
Major illness/injury	53
Marriage	50
Being made redundant	47
Marital reconciliation	45
Retirement	45
Major change in health or behaviour of family member	44
Pregnancy	40
Sexual Difficulties	39
Adding to family (birth, adoption, elderly parents moving in)	39
Major business readjustments	39
Major change in financial state	38
Death of a close friend	36
Change of work	36
Arguments with spouse	35
Assuming a mortgage	31
Foreclosure on mortgage or loan	30
More job responsibility	29
Children leaving home	29
In-law trouble	29
Outstanding personal achievement	28
Wife starting or leaving work	26
Starting or leaving school	26

Major change in living conditions	25
Changing personal habits	24
Trouble with the boss	23
Major change in working hours or conditions	20
Moving house	20
Moving school	20
Major change in recreation	19
Major change in church activities	19
Major change in social activities	18
Assuming a small loan	17
Major change in sleeping habits	16
Increased or reduced family get-togethers	15
Major change in eating habits	15
Holidays	13
Christmas	12
Minor violations of the law	11

Score (over the last year):

   Over 300: you have an 80% chance of developing a serious illness within the next two years.

   150–300: you have a 50% chance of developing a serious illness within the next two years.

   Below 150: you have a 33% chance of developing a serious illness within the next two years.

Don't be too alarmed by these figures. Health is more than a matter of statistics. The value of this rating lies more in getting us to realise *when* we are likely to be particularly stressed and need to take it easy and relax and be good to ourselves than in scaring us to death.

Stress Can Kill You

As Selye pointed out, stress is not always bad. It can be stimulating and some people get high on it, sometimes quite literally as in mountain climbing or racing fast cars. Successfully meeting challenges gives us a feeling of satisfaction, that Selye calls "eustress." It can be a spur to achievement, and sometimes actually speeds up a cure when someone is ill. And of course we all have our different tolerance levels; what is stressful for some may be less stressful or not stressful at all for others.

But unrelieved stress that goes on for too long or is too much to handle is almost certainly the biggest single cause of illness, whether this manifests on the physical or the mental/emotional plane. It has been estimated that as many as 70% of patients waiting in their GP's surgery every day will be there because they are experiencing stress. In a recent study by Dr. Norman Beale it was found that Tredundancy (or the threat of it) led to a 20% increase in visits to GPs and a 60% rise in hospital visits.

The severity of the malady that can follow in the wake of too much stress is in the lap of the gods. The Common Cold Research Unit in Salisbury in the early eighties came up with the fact that those most likely to catch a cold were those who had recently experienced major changes along the lines of the Holmes/Rahe ratings, e.g., bereavement, marriage, divorce, retirement and job loss. We have already seen the correlation between loss and bereavement and the onset of cancer. The world's biggest killer today—the coronary—is also very likely caused more by stress than any other single factor such as too much cholesterol, obesity or smoking.

Drs. Roffosenman and Friedman checked the blood-cholesterol levels of a group of accountants over a six-month period, starting at the New Year. They discovered that the levels rose as the start of the financial year in April approached, and fell again after work-loads returned to normal and the pressure was off. The accountants' diets and life-styles had not changed during this six month period—only the amount of stress to which they were exposed.

We are continually being exposed to stress, not only in our personal lives but also environmentally. Polluted air, noisy traffic, urban violence—or the fear of it—pace and competition all add their toll, and every day for those of us who live in cities.

In 1962, research conducted among a small, quiet Italian community in Roseto, Pennsylvania, revealed a lower incidence of heart disease and less than half the death rate from this cause than among the inhabitants of neighbouring towns.

Some of the inhabitants had left to seek work in neighbouring cities. When they were traced, the researchers found that these urbanised Rosetans now had mortality rates closer to the general average. These findings were borne out by the investigation made by the Harvard School of Nutrition in 1982 into the health of nearly 600 Irishmen who emigrated to Boston. Their brothers remained in Ireland, a country where people eat more saturated fat (especially butter) than in almost any other country in the world. Those who went to America to find work in a big city enjoyed a healthier diet—yet eventually they developed more heart trouble than their brothers who had stayed at home in rural Ireland.

Stress and AIDS

In an article in the San Francisco newspaper *The Bay Area Reporter* on September 29th, 1983, psychotherapist Jeff M. Leiphart expressed the view that stress is a key factor in causing AIDS.

Dr. Leiphart had spent eighteen months administering therapy to 26 men diagnosed with AIDS or AIDS related conditions (ARC). Each of these men showed what he called an unresolved "emotional urgency" dating back to early childhood and relating to survival. In other words, none of them had ever felt *safe*. It is hardly surprising that homosexuals (especially male homosexuals) should feel unsafe in a society that at best tolerates them, at worst discriminates against and condemns them. As many have to live with the constant threat of invalidation and disapproval for being oneself—anxiety about "exposure," being judged, even being physically attacked—it is not surprising that their immune system should be continually on "red alert." Selye described how the powerful hormones released by the stress response can damage the body's nervous system, organs and immune system. The process happens like this: the hypothalamus in the brain activates the pituitary gland to release hormones that govern the endocrine system. The adrenals then go into action, releasing adrenalin and corticosteroids. Chronically elevated cortisol levels due to unrelieved stress (as in the case of Leiphart's patients) will suppress the immune system. It reduces the number of T helper cells, increases T suppressors (see page 6), inhibits the production of killer cells and reduces interferon, a first line of defence against invading viruses.

It would seem therefore that, far from being a "Gay Plague," AIDS is a plague visited upon gays by a society blocked from respecting differences and short on compassion, and that they are more sinned against than sinning. Medical clairvoyant, author and journalist Caroline Myss has suggested that susceptibility to AIDS is the outcome of the "victim consciousness" of those who perceive themselves to be outcasts, and points to those who are in the high risk groups: male homosexuals, Haitians, prostitutes, drug abusers and inhabitants of Africa, the most victimised part of our planet.

ILLNESS AS LACK OF LOVE

We have already seen the connection between experiencing loss of love and the onset of catastrophic illness such as cancer. It is as if we can lose our will to live without our partner, or at some deep, subconscious level, decide to follow them. We can, almost literally, die of a broken heart. It is significant that the thymus which plays such a key role in our immune system is situated near the heart, which has always been seen as the shrine of feeling.

This perception that life is not worth living without love is perhaps not unfounded. We need it to survive. It is the *lingua franca* of this planet, the only language that is universally understood. Babies understand it, so do animals and plants. Without it they do not flourish, and can wither and die. But even more important than to be on the receiving end of love from others is to love ourselves. Self-hatred is self-destructive; it suppresses the immune system as nothing else does. At least if we are attacked from the outside, we have the option of defending ourselves. When the persecutor is within, we are psychologically defenceless—and, as always, what goes on inside the body mirrors our psychic reality. My own experience over the years as a counsellor and therapist is that very few people love themselves. The bottom line with almost everybody I have ever worked with is "I am not good enough." From this basic, conditioned misperception is spawned most of the unhappiness that plagues us. It damages our mental, emotional and bodily health, inhibits us from freely expressing ourselves and kills all joy in relating to our fellows, to whom we will tend to relate in a distorted fashion—rating them either as low as we rate ourselves or as impossibly high above us. By contrast, as Louise Hay puts it, "Happiness is feeling good about yourself." Loving and experiencing being loved not only makes us feel good, it actually *does* us good, notably by stimulating the all-important thymus that plays such a crucial role in maintaining our immune system in peak condition.

Lawrence LeShan, a New York psychologist and author, once examined the psychological characteristics of 250 cancer patients and came up with a "cancer profile." As well as experiencing a sense of loss (which we have come to associate with cancer already) they all suffered from feelings of self-hatred, inability to come to their own defence if attacked, and tension in relationship to their parents.

In the case of those who feel victimised by society, introjecting social disapproval of their life-style would be even more hazardous to their health than the simple fact of prejudice and intolerance. Attempting to find relief from the depression that comes from having a low self-image could lead in some cases (though of course not all) to self-destructive behaviour like abuse of drugs and alcohol and/or promiscuity (which is nothing more than the compulsive pursuit of love by someone who deep down thinks he or she is unworthy of it). There is then more likelihood of VD resulting in an intake of more antibiotics, and more stress on an immune system already at risk . . .

The Healing Power of Love

Now for the good news, love heals—and more than anything else.

I am convinced that unconditional love is the most powerful known stimulant of the immune system. If I told patients to raise their blood levels of immune globulins or killer T cells, no one would know how. But if I can teach them to love themselves and other fully, the same changes happen automatically. The truth is, love heals. (Bernie Siegel, Assistant Clinical Professor of Surgery at Yale Medical School. The quote is from his book, *Love, Medicine and Miracles*.)

Even watching love movies helps, as shown by Harvard psychologists David McClelland and Carol Kirshnit in 1982, who found that watching such movies increased levels of immunoglobulin-A in the saliva. Immunoglobulin-A is our first line of defence against colds and other viral diseases. The same researchers found that a documentary on the work of Mother Teresa produced an immediate and appreciable rise of immunoglobulin levels in the saliva of viewers, quite unrelated to their conscious like or dislike of the saintly nun.

It seems that even just thinking about loving experiences of the past is healing. According to Dr. David McClelland, dwelling on the positive experiences of loving and being loved also raised immunoglobulin levels. But in case you are worried about what you might be doing to yourself by exposing yourself to a nightly ration of horror and violence on television, be reassured by the fact that researchers found that being shown a film about Hitler elicited no response one way or the other. Even if it had, you could always take prophylactic action by stroking your cat while watching the programme. Dr. Aaron Katche of Pennsylvania University has found that petting an animal to which one is bonded leads to lower blood pressure. Between 1975 and 1977 he followed up the progress of 932 coronary patients for one year after their discharge from hospital. Of the 53 pet owners amongst them only 3 had died, compared to 11 of the 39 without pets.

two

NEGATIVITY AND ILLNESS

Just as love heals, so harbouring negative feelings can make us ill. In a survey similar to LeShan's (page 14), Carl and Stephanie Simonton discovered that the typical cancer patient evinces a strong tendency to hold resentment and a reluctance to forgive, together with an inclination towards self-pity and, perhaps predictably in view of this, a poor ability to develop and maintain meaningful long-term relationships.

A doctor at the University of Amsterdam named Wouter Oosterhuis investigated 500 patients complaining of pain for which there was no obvious physical cause. Of 331 who owned to aggressive feelings, 329 suffered with pains in the neck, nine out of ten who experienced fear had abdominal pains, and six out of ten with lower back pains were experiencing despair.

To quote Bernie Siegel again: "The simple truth is, happy people generally don't get sick. One's attitude to oneself is the single most important factor in healing or staying well. Those who are at peace with themselves and their immediate surroundings have far fewer serious illnesses than those who are not." He quotes Dr. Ellerbroek who collected 57 well-documented cancer "miracles." In each case, the cure followed the patient's conscious decision to give up their anger and depression. From that point, their tumours started to shrink.

This echoes the experience of Louise Hay who healed herself of vaginal cancer in six months by choosing to let go of her long-held resentment at her treatment as an abused child. She intuited that acid thoughts created acid blood that was eating away at her body—so she let go of these thoughts. She considers that the most self-destructive feelings we can harbour are those of guilt, criticism and resentment. In *A Course in Miracles*, Helen Schucman goes as far as to claim that *all* illness stems from a lack of forgiveness.

By contrast, the benefits of enjoying ourselves and having a good laugh have long been suspected. As far back as the second century AD, Galen had observed that it was depressed women who got breast cancer, not cheerful ones. That "laughter is the best medicine" is at last beginning to be taken seriously by the medical profession, especially in the French-speaking world. In 1986 a symposium was held in Toronto for doctors, nurses and therapists on the healing power of laughter.

In his best-selling book *Anatomy of an Illness*, Norman Cousins told us how he healed himself of the crippling and "incurable" ankylosing spondylitis (a disease of the body's connective tissues) after having been given one chance in 500 of survival. He cured himself with high doses of vitamin C and good belly-laughs at videos of *Candid Camera* and old Marx Brothers films.

French researchers have found that laughers are less prone to ulcers and other digestive disorders. According to Dr. Pierre Dacher, laughter improves circulation, speeds tissue healing and stabilises many bodily functions. Sir William Osler called it "the music of life"; Norman Cousins, "internal jogging."

To enjoy ourselves is one of the most prophylactic things we can do for our health. When we are doing so, we are flowing with our energy, relaxing, unstressed, more alive, feeling good—and our bodies respond to our messages that life is indeed worth living and we want more of it. In fact, the shortest cut to self-healing is to deliberately cultivate this "feeling good" by any means we know how, and as often as we can each day.

Many of the techniques described in this book do that, e.g., choosing to think positive rather than negative thoughts, validating ourselves through affirmations, treating ourselves to massage and light exercise, etc. Make it a golden rule when you are ill to find things that give you pleasure, to do only things that you enjoy doing, and to give yourself permission not to do anything because you feel you *should*.

THE POWER OF THE MIND

Sir William Osler, the Canadian physician and medical historian, remarked once that the outcome of TB had more to do with what was going on in the patient's mind than in his lungs. He seems to be echoing Hippocrates, who said that he would rather know what sort of person has a disease than what sort of disease a person has.

Side by side with our growing awareness of the paramount importance of the immune system in maintaining health is our increasing recognition of the part played by the mind and feelings in both causing and healing illness. Together they are producing a quiet revolution in medicine as the new science of psychoimmunology begins to emerge. Bacteria, viruses and tumours are undoubtedly present, but it is coming to be seen that their power and malignancy are more and more dependent on what is going on in their host. The strength or weakness of an immune system is in turn affected by what we think, feel, say and do—even, as we have seen, by what we choose to look at.

"Years of experience have taught me," says Bernie Siegel, "that cancer and indeed nearly all diseases are psychosomatic." Dr. Edward Bach went even further. He claimed that *all* disease was a manifestation of underlying negative states of mind. After working in London for 20 years as a consultant bacteriologist and homoeopath, Bach gave up his lucrative Harley Street practice in order to devote all his time to discovering plant remedies which would heal illness by countering these negative mental states. The 39 Bach Flower Remedies (listed in Part II see pages 109–112) are each very specifically geared to treating a particular negative state, such as guilt, fear or panic.

As long as 50 years ago, in experiments at the University of Vienna, it was demonstrated that cold sores could be made to erupt in patients under hypnosis simply by reminding them of painful experiences in their past. Whatever goes on in the mind and the feelings is mirrored immediately in the body. Measurements of various bodily functions have been correlated with emotional states in a system called "sentic cycles" by a psychophysiological researcher named Dr. Manfred Clynes. These show clearly that negativity churns up not only the mind and the emotions, but the body as well. Dr. Clynes gets his subjects to work themselves up into an emotional state by imagining situations likely to induce it. The prescribed emotions (which he calls "sentic states"), in the required sequence are:

> no emotion
> anger
> hate
> grief
> love
> sex
> joy
> reverence.

At a given signal, while in each of these states, the subject presses what looks like a piano key, which records the finger pressure on a chart. At the same time the subject's bodily functions are also being monitored and recorded.

Clyne's system is a form of biofeedback; a "feeding back" to us of information showing what goes on in our bodies when we think or feel certain things. Thoughts create feelings in the body, which then prepares to act on them. The body has no way of differentiating between what is subjective and what is objective, what is, for example, "imagined danger" and what is "real danger." The same physiological chain reactions will be activated, in the direction of arousal, what is often called "fight or flight," or what Benson has termed the "relaxation response."

Other biofeedback systems (e.g., the "Mind Mirror" invented by Geoffrey G. Blundell) show us the brain activity associated with these states. When we are awake, thinking, doing, concentrating, the usual rhythm of our brainwaves is predominantly on the Beta frequency. This means that the electrical activity of our brains varies within the range of 14 to 26 times a second (usually measured as cycles per second indicated by the symbol Hz). The more anxious, angry or worried we are (i.e., the more under stress) the higher we go into Beta. What happens when we relax? Our brainwaves slow down to the lower frequency of 8 to 13 Hz that we call Alpha. If we slow down even more, (below 7 Hz) we enter the Theta wavelength, the half-asleep or dreaming state. When we are in deep and dreamless sleep, our brainwaves have slowed down to between ½ and 4 Hz and we are in Delta.

The prototype for the Mind Mirror was first used on one of C. Maxwell Cade's courses in meditation and relaxation in June 1976. He was a Fellow of the Royal Society of Medicine who had become interested in investigating the brainwaves that he saw on EEG (electro-encephalogram) tracings of patients in hospitals. Together with Geoffrey Blundell, an engineer, he produced a two-channel portable machine which could analyse signals from the left and right hemispheres of the brain and display them on a monitor as a pattern of little red lights. The perfected model is still being used on similar (and healing) courses currently being run in London by Maxwell Cade's widow, Isabel. If you are interested in trying biofeedback for yourself you can contact her at the telephone number listed in the Appendix.

On pages 21–24 are reproduced examples of how brainwave patterns show up on the Mind Mirror. The numbers down the outside of the diagrams show the frequency, ranging from 38 Hz in Beta down to 0.75 in Delta. The small numbers along the horizontal lines indicate the amplitude of the signal (the 1–16 figures measured in millionths of a volt). Movement of the position of the black dot away from the centre towards the left shows the degree of left hemisphere activity, and the movement towards the right, activity of the right hemisphere.

Diagrams 1 and 2 show "Alpha blocking," the apprehensive or unsure response of the average person to first being connected to a biofeedback machine. Beta is predominant in both, the subject in diagram 2 producing the excessive Beta

DIAGRAM 1: Beta States

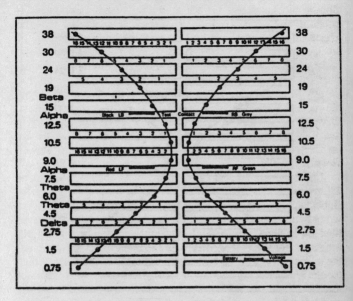

Diagrams 1, 2, 3 and 4 show the Mind Mirror (see pages 19–20). They are taken from Geoffrey Blundell's *The Meaning of EEG: A study in depth of brainwave patterns and their significance.*

typical of the "fight or flight" response. Diagrams 3 and 4 show Alpha states in which the subject has "switched off" involvement with the external world and is experiencing the "relaxation response."

It is when we stay too long in Beta that we are in for trouble. Not only because prolonged stress in the form of thinking, doing and worrying too much undermines the immune system, but because we will also tend to get fatigued and be more accident prone. Daily sessions of deep relaxation are prophylactic; relaxing into Alpha recharges batteries as nothing else can—not even, it has been proved, sleep. It repairs the ravages of stress at a deep level and strengthens the immune system.

We instinctively take to our beds whenever we feel ill be-

DIAGRAM 2: Beta States

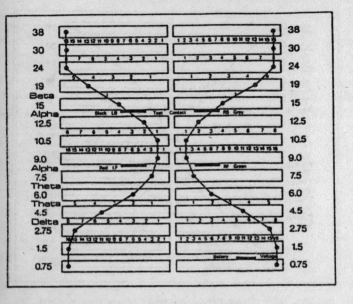

cause our inner wisdom tells us that rest is the biggest single factor in restoring us to health. But merely resting the body is not sufficient unless our minds also are at rest and our hearts at peace. We can be lying down yet all the while be tormented by thoughts that won't switch off or feelings that cause us anguish. The prone position of our bodies will be belied by the inner churning up that is following in the wake of this inner turmoil. We will get no real peace until we learn how to facilitate our own relaxation response—and at levels including mental, emotional and spiritual, not just physical. This is why meditation and yoga are such powerful tools for healing. Once you get the hang of them, they get you down to Alpha fast.

In 1961, in New Delhi, Dr. B. K. Anand reported the same increases of Alpha brainwave activity in yoga practitioners as

DIAGRAM 3: Alpha States

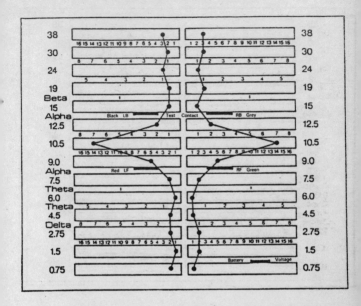

were discovered five years later in Zen meditators by Drs. Kasamatsu and Hirai of the University of Tokyo.

In 1976, Gurucharan Singh Lhals, founder of Boston's Kundalini Research Institute confirmed that regular meditation and yoga improve our immunity, causing blood levels of three important immune system hormones to increase by as much as 100%. His findings were confirmed by Alberto Villoldo of San Francisco State College, who in 1980 reported improved white cell response and improved efficiency of hormone response to stress after regular meditation and visualisation.

But the importance of the Alpha state for healing is crucial for another reason. While we are in Alpha, with slowed down thought processes and a deeply relaxed body, miracles of healing can happen. We become much more susceptible to autosuggestion. We can "plant" healing suggestions in the form

DIAGRAM 4: Alpha States

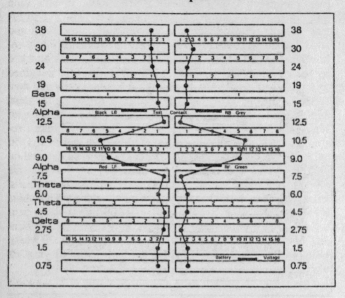

of positive verbal affirmations or healing images that will be immediately acted on by the body, often with spectacular results.

Healing Images

The work of Carl Simonton, radiation oncologist and medical director of the Cancer Counselling and Research Center at Fort Worth, Texas, is now well known from his bestselling book *Getting Well Again*. Simonton first became interested in the power of the mind to affect the course of disease as a result of treating female cancer patients with radiation therapy. He was struck by the fact that those women who *anticipated* the worst *suffered* the worst side effects.

Simonton first used visualisation therapy in 1971 on a 60-

year-old man afflicted with advanced throat cancer. The patient was asked to participate in a programme of relaxation and visualisation carried out three times a day for five to fifteen minutes, on awakening in the morning, after lunch and at night before going to sleep. When he was sufficiently relaxed, he was asked to visualise the cancer cells being attacked by the radiation therapy he was also receiving. He imagined tiny bullets of energy destroying the malignant cells and then created a picture of his body's white cells removing the dead and dying cancer cells. The visualisation process ended with seeing the tumour shrink in size and a picture of himself restored to radiant health. It worked. The patient gained weight, and felt better and stronger. Two months later, he showed no sign of cancer. The sequel to this success story was that the patient went on to use the technique to improve his arthritis, smoothing the joint surfaces in his mind to the point where his symptoms had decreased sufficiently for him to enjoy fishing again. Now thoroughly confident, he went on to cure himself of the sexual impotence that had lasted over 20 years. Using visualisation, after only two weeks he was enjoying sex once again.

This is not an isolated cure. The survival rate of Simonton's patients is twice the national average. These techniques are now being used with equal success in Cancer Help Centres in Britain (notably at Bristol) and are beginning to interest the medical establishment. At the time of writing I have just received a letter from Pat Pilkington, co-founder and Director of the Bristol Cancer Help Centre, telling me that they have been approached by the National Health Service (from the Hammersmith Hospital in London) to help them set up a Cancer Help Centre department in their Oncology Unit. As Pat put it, "This is a tremendous breakthrough in the thinking of orthodox medicine and we are all extremely excited by it. This event has caused quite a stir and we have been inundated by visits from radio, television and journalists."

The power of mental images is matched by the power of words. It behoves us to become aware of the danger of crying "wolf!" too often, for example, with hypochondria. We can actually invite illness by fearing it. Our body in its obedient innocence accepts whatever messages we feed into our mind-computer and obligingly comes up with the experience which matches it. To put it another way: the universe gives us more of what we are experiencing. It makes more real any reality we choose to create for ourselves. Tremendously respectful of our freedom, life supplies more ''juice'' to manifest on the physical plane whatever we are choosing to believe is true about ourselves. We literally do create our own reality, our own experience, for better or for worse—which is why miracles, or disasters happen to us.

It is an awe-inspiring thought that, moment to moment, we are creating our future by what we think, feel and say. What we tell ourselves is supremely important for our health.

We shall be learning in Part II how to create new, healthy realities for ourselves by means of affirmations: affirming the ways of being that work for us rather than against us; creating new life-affirming mental patterns to replace the stale and negative ones that have made us ill; planting seeds of positivity deep in our subconscious that soon (if we have faith) begin to blossom and bear fruit in, at best, a restoration to health and, at the very least, joy and peace of mind.

As Louise Hay proved for herself and is proving daily to many others, among them people with AIDS, ''*dissolving mental patterns dissolves disease.*''

As Simonton confirms, the agent of change (together with love) is *belief*. In a study of 152 cancer patients he established that the positive attitude towards treatment was a better predictor of response to treatment than was the severity of the disease. Put another way, this means that anything can be healed—*if you believe it can*. And anything can be an agent of healing if you have enough faith in it, from prayer to placebos, from crystals to crucifixes.

| three |

ENERGY AND ILLNESS

We intuitively grasp the connection between vitality and good health. We talk of "lacking energy," of being "run down," of feeling "drained," or of having "overdone it" when explaining to a friend why we think we caught that cold or the flu. Fatigue is often the first sign that we are "coming down" with something and is a symptom of many illnesses. If we equate the state of our immune system with the more homely term "resistance" we would not be far wrong. We understand instinctively that we have to "keep our strength up," for example with nourishing food and adequate rest, if we are to stay well or get well.

Thinking in terms of energy is central to the holistic view of health and the healing process, and is found in cultures besides our own. In yoga this vital energy is called *prana*, in acupuncture *chi*, in martial arts *ki*, by Polynesians *mana*, by American Indians, *orenda*.

Virtually the whole of what we term "alternative therapy" is based on a view of human beings—indeed, all life—as energy processes. And, when you come to think of it, it makes sense. Consider what we are doing when we breathe in the air, ingest food, talk with or make love to each other. We are taking in energy, converting it into other forms and putting it out again. In a very basic sense, we are all energy transformers. In describing how we are putting out this energy we almost seem to be describing electricity; someone is being "positive" or "negative," he is "dynamic," she is "radiant."

Kirlian Photography

That the existence of body energy is a reality can be shown objectively. It can actually be photographed. A Russian electrician named Semyon Kirlian and his wife, Valentina, invented an aluminium plate to which a high-frequency field is delivered. This plate is covered by another plate of glass over which goes the film. The subject for the "Kirlian effect" places his or her hand on the film, which is protected from salt in the skin by a piece of plastic. A pressure gauge ensures that the hand pressure remains constant. Using this technique, one ends up with the imprint of the person's hand surrounded by patterns and colours—the energy field or aura. Kirlian discovered that when he was ill, the energy-field photographed around his hand became blurred and faint, while that of his wife (who was well) remained clear and bright. Since then research has been undertaken in Russia and, in the 1970s, in the West. It has been shown that Kirlian photography can be used successfully for the diagnosis of certain illnesses before the symptoms become overt.

Biorhythms

That there is a connection between low-energy states and "disease"—of whatever variety—is indisputable, as is the fact that our energy-levels change according to a very definite rhythm. According to the theory of biorhythms each of us is influenced by three biological cycles which begin at birth and continue for the rest of our lives. The physical cycle lasts 23 days and influences our resistance to disease, strength, endurance and eye-hand coordination. The emotional cycle is 28 days long and influences our emotional states, e.g., optimism/pessimism, passion/coldness, elation/depression. The intellectual cycle lasts 33 days and influences our alertness, speed of learning, reasoning ability, accuracy of computation and memory.

At the moment of birth, according to biorhythm theory, each

cycle starts at a zero point and begins to rise in a positive phase during which the energies and abilities are high. After reaching a positive peak, each cycle then gradually declines, crossing its zero point midway through its period, (i.e., 11 ½ days for the physical, 14 days for the emotional, and 16 ½ days for the intellectual). The remainder of the cycle is a negative phase, during which our energies and capabilities are reduced. The most unstable times are the ''critical days'' in each cycle, when the cycle crosses its zero point, changing from positive to negative and from negative to positive. During these critical days, the abilities vary wildly, from extremely high to extremely low. You may make brilliant discoveries or disastrous logical errors on intellectually critical days. You may be overflowing with energy or feeling totally drained on physically critical days. You may impulsively propose marriage or impulsively quit your job on emotionally critical days.

A family member suffered a heart attack (fortunately a mild one) on October 6th last year. After his recovery and return to work he, quite by chance, happened to have access to a chart of his biorhythms. Browsing through it (somewhat sceptically) he was struck by the fact that October 6th had been a critical day physically for him. It also happened to have been a particularly busy day at work where he was under extra pressure. It would appear that stress is particularly lethal when it coincides with a ''bad day,'' biorhythmically speaking.

Biorhythms can be charted for each individual. The first biorhythm calculator was produced by the Swiss in 1927 and they have used them (as have the Japanese and the Americans) in factories for safety, in hospitals for calculating the best time (for both patients and surgeons) for carrying out surgery, and in the selection of national gymnastic teams for high-level performance.

Our energy levels, then, go up and down. The flow of our energy can also be blocked or out of balance, and, for the ''alternative therapist,'' this is the true cause of illness. He or she will therefore note but not be as interested in treating the manifestation of such blockage or imbalance (i.e., the patient's symptoms) so much as the underlying disharmony that has given rise to them. The acupuncturist, for example, will work

directly with needles and *moxa* on certain points along the
energy meridians to balance and redirect the flow of *chi* (energy). (*Moxa* is a technique used in acupuncture to promote
energy flow along a meridian, as an adjunct to treatment with
needles. A tiny cone of moxa or common mugwort is placed
on the needle over the selected acupuncture point, and then
lit. It is extinguished just before it comes into contact with the
skin of the patient.) And the homoeopath will delve into the
Materia Medica (book of remedies) to try to come up with
just the right remedy to stimulate the body's vitality to restore
itself to harmony and balance.

The effectiveness of allopathic (or traditional) medicine in
crisis situations is undoubted. Where acupuncture and homoeopathy score over it is in that they are able to "catch"
illness in its subtle, pre-symptomatic stage and, hopefully,
avert it. Unless you can present your doctor with something
that shows up on an X ray or some other means of identifying
organic malfunction, he is virtually helpless. And yet all illness
begins on subtle energy levels before it goes on to manifest
on the grosser material plane, i.e., the body. Just consider how
before you went down with that bout of flu you started to feel
"off." If you were sufficiently in touch with your own process
you would have remarked a vague feeling of being "below
par," perhaps slightly depressed or irritable, looking a little
wan and lacking energy.

As a medical student, Sir Hans Selye noted how, in the early
stages of illness, the syndrome of "just being sick" always
made its appearance first: vague aches, upset stomachs, feeling
unwell and so on. His teachers, predictably, were not interested in these non-specific symptoms. But, years later, Selye
was to suggest that they are significant as registering the
body's first alarm signals. The price for ignoring them would
depend on the strength of the body's immune system (or, as
he called it, "adaptation energy") to handle the subsequent,
if unchecked, progression on to more overt and specific symptom manifestation. This symptom manifestation is really the
end of a long process. One just does not "suddenly" fall ill,
even though it may appear that way.

Dr. Peter Nixon, consultant in cardiology at Charing Cross
Hospital, together with Dr. David Peters, a GP practising in

Hayes, have been stressing the importance of directing attention to bodily signals when we are in this nether land between being well and not yet having brewed up specific illness.

John Davidson puts this general "unwellness" down to the dissonance created in cellular, molecular, sub-atomic, emotional and mental energies. In his book *Subtle Energy* (see Further Reading), he suggests that whether it is modern conventional medicine and surgery or more esoteric forms of healing, the applied therapy does no more than rearrange the energy patterns of the body, mind and emotions in order to create harmony and health.

SYMPTOM MANIFESTATION

Disease, then, is always preceded by "dis-ease"—by a disharmony in our more subtle energies (or the aura as discovered by Kirlian) that, if we are sufficiently in tune with ourselves, can be experienced as some sort of malaise or tension in our consciousness. There is a part of us, our inner wisdom, that tells us when things are not quite right. But we have to be listening to its voice in order to hear it. Too often we are too busy, too deafened by what's going on outside us to become aware of what's going on closer to home. So we don't heed the messages to ease up, to conserve the energy, to nourish ourselves better, to let go of what needs to be let go of, and we continue to pile on the stress until overt symptoms develop.

Why the body manifests symptoms in particular sites is not always clear. Sometimes there seems to be a literal connection between the form of stress one is under and the part of the body that is experiencing pain. We can often trace a connection between, for example, a "slipped disc" or lower back pain and feeling that one is not supported enough in one's life; and between aching shoulder muscles and feeling that one has to carry too much responsibility. The symptoms seem to be metaphors, to be reflecting on the bodily plane what is going on with us on the psychic plane: the function of the back is to support; and shoulders are associated with carrying burdens.

These metaphors have passed into ordinary speech. We talk

of someone being "brokenhearted," of being "eaten away
with envy or resentment," of being "choked with grief."
Someone who is ungiving we may refer to as "constipated,"
another we experience as never having any energy we may
call "anaemic." Resistance to a person's communication or
behaviour can make us tighten up our muscles in a way that
makes us experience our interaction literally as a "pain in the
neck"—or even a "pain in the ass"—which is then what we
may call them. We can make ourselves myopic or even blind
if there are things in our lives we do not want to have to look
at, or deaf if we feel threatened by what we might hear. It has
even been suggested that there are no such things as "accidents." If we want to avoid doing something enough, but feel
we have no honourable way of doing so, or have a sufficiently
strong self-destructive pattern or need for punishment in our
subconscious, somehow we will find a way, albeit unconsciously, to sabotage our conscious intentions. Guilt always
manifests as pain in some way, self-hatred which is anger
turned inwards, as depression.

Miasms

The founder of homoeopathy, the German physician Samuel
Hahnemann (1755–1843) considered that there were certain
basic vibrational patterns of disease that he termed *miasms*.
These *miasms* are acquired by various contagions or traumas
or inherited from our parents, or caused by levels of toxic
pollution in our food or environment. A *miasm* is essentially
a built-in disease pattern, energy disharmony or imbalance,
which decides the types of illnesses we are likely to get. The
term is used to describe a chronic state of ill-health where the
pattern has become fixed.

   According to homoeopathic theory there are three major inherited *miasms; psora, sycosis*, and *syphilis*. The characteristic
of *psora* is underfunctioning on all planes, physical, mental
and emotional; that of *sycosis* manifests as overfunctioning;
while *syphilis* is associated with degeneration. The sorts of
symptoms that go with each would include dryness of mucus
membranes, skin eruptions, fibroids (*psora*), ulcers, venereal

disease—especially gonorrhea—growths, mental illness (*sy-cosis*), degenerative diseases (syphilis) not associated with the disease itself. What this means is that we are pre-disposed to certain types of illness rather than others and indicates why certain types of illnesses tend to run in families.

The Chakras

Probably the most sophisticated model for trying to understand why disease hits us where it does is to be found in the eastern theory of the chakras. The seven chakras are energy centres in the body associated with endocrine glands and nerve clusters. (See the chart on page 34.)

The first, or root chakra is situated at the base of the spine, at the tailbone or coccyx and controls the adrenals. The energy mediated by this chakra is to do with survival, as one would expect from the fact that it is through the release of adrenalin that we are activated into "fight or flight." The second chakra, located just above the genitals, is associated with the gonads and is the "sex chakra." The third chakra is in the solar plexus and is the centre we come from when we experience "gut feelings" or exercise our personal power. It is linked with the pancreas. The fourth chakra on the cardiac plexus is the heart centre, where all the lower chakras are integrated into love, which is harmony. The thymus, the original central activator of the entire endocrine system and immune system (situated at the top of the sternum below the Adam's apple) is intimately associated with it. The fifth chakra, associated with the thyroid, is the throat chakra, the seat of self-expression. The sixth chakra is in the centre of the forehead, and relates to the pituitary. It governs our intuition and is the headquarters of our mind and soul in the waking state. The seventh chakra, or brain chakra, is at the top of the head. Linked with the pineal gland, it represents our connection with what is beyond the limited consciousness of the body and allows us to express ourselves on high spiritual levels.

Each chakra is to do with a specific area in our lives and patterns of experiencing. If we are experiencing stress in a particular area, tension ("dis-ease") will start to come through

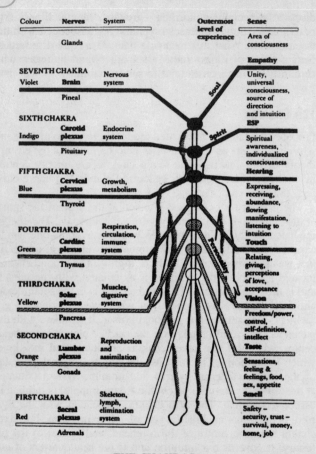

Colour	Nerves	System		Outermost level of experience	Sense
	Glands				Area of consciousness
					Empathy
SEVENTH CHAKRA	**Brain**	Nervous system	Soul		Unity, universal consciousness, source of direction and intuition
Violet	Pineal				ESP
SIXTH CHAKRA	**Carotid plexus**	Endocrine system	Spirit		Spiritual awareness, individualized consciousness
Indigo	Pituitary				Hearing
FIFTH CHAKRA	**Cervical plexus**	Growth, metabolism			Expressing, receiving, abundance, flowing manifestation, listening to intuition
Blue	Thyroid				Touch
FOURTH CHAKRA	**Cardiac plexus**	Respiration, circulation, immune system	Personality		Relating, giving, perceptions of love, acceptance
Green	Thymus				Vision
THIRD CHAKRA	**Solar plexus**	Muscles, digestive system			Freedom/power, control, self-definition, intellect
Yellow	Pancreas				Taste
SECOND CHAKRA	**Lumbar plexus**	Reproduction and assimilation			Sensations, feeling & feelings, food, sex, appetite
Orange	Gonads				Smell
FIRST CHAKRA	**Sacral plexus**	Skeleton, lymph, elimination system			Safety – security, trust – survival, money, home, job
Red	Adrenals				

THE CHAKRAS

on that chakra wave-length and, if not handled at source, will tend to manifest in symptoms in the part or parts of the body governed by that chakra. Thus, as we have already seen in the case of Leiphart's AIDS patients, anxiety about survival (first chakra) and feeling unsafe in a hostile world is, over a long period, likely to exhaust the adrenals with consequent damage to the immune system—as is also stress on the thymus (fourth or heart chakra) ensuing from perceptions of being unlovable to and unaccepted by oneself or others. The victim consciousness described by Caroline Myss (page 13) is the preoccupation of the third chakra, to do with personal power and governing muscles and the digestive system.

That imbalance in at least three of the chakras are probably involved in the onset of AIDS would perhaps explain the many-sidedness of its symptomatology: the variety of opportunistic infections stemming from an impaired immune system, such as *pneumocystis carinii* (a form of pnemonia), Kaposi's sarcoma, candida and parasitic infections of the bowel.

We have also seen how cancer is very much associated with unexpressed feeling, and lack of emotional outlet is common amongst cancer patients. This would manifest in a blockage of energy coming through the fifth or throat chakra associated with the endocrine system. It has been said that it is the "nice" people who get cancer. The 1986 study of 2,163 women reported that women most likely to develop breast cancer are those who are reluctant to show emotion and are withdrawn and less competitive.

By contrast, psychologist Leonard Zerogatis found in a study of 35 women with breast cancer that the long-term survivors were the ones who were judged to have a bad relationship with their doctors in that they expressed themselves freely and asked a lot of questions.

Caroline Myss has stressed the importance for women, particularly, to speak up for themselves and to free themselves from dependence on their menfolk if they are to avoid disorders of their reproductive system arising from feeling disempowered in intimate relationships, which leads to imbalance in the second chakra. (G. F. Solomon too has linked arthritis in women with renunciation of or loss of independence.)

The reason why some people are particularly vulnerable to catching venereal disease while others go unscathed may well be explainable in terms of energy blockage in this sex chakra due to unresolved feelings of guilt about sex.

The chakra theory may also provide the answer to our question about the greater susceptibility of men than women to heart disease. The heart is the centre of feeling, and in our culture women are permitted to express their feelings more easily than men. Once again illness can be a metaphor: what is a coronary but a constriction of the heart?

After prayer and the laying on of hands (which Dr. Bernard Grad, an associate professor of psychiatry at McGill University, considers channels an actual healing force that can be measured under laboratory conditions), healing through the chakras is probably the technique most widely practised among non-medical healers. In part II we shall be seeing how to do this for ourselves.

four

THE MEANING OF ILLNESS

When illness strikes, apparently out of the blue, it brings us up with a jolt, and if it is severe enough, stops us carrying on as usual. And perhaps this is precisely what it is intended to do: it is its biological function and *raison d'être*.

Illness and the Psyche

Jung pointed out that the development of neurosis is the attempt by the Unconscious to compensate for a too-one-sided Ego-consciousness that is producing imbalance in the psyche. It is a sign that we are not seeing things we should be seeing, not allowing change in areas we should be changing, and not accepting things in ourselves that should be accepted if we are to progress towards wholeness and become more and more truly ourselves.

Inconvenient and perhaps even distressing symptoms do in fact have a purpose. They are the attempts of the self-regulating psyche to heal itself, and point us in the direction of the necessary changes that need to be made in our lives and way of thinking. Freeing blocked energy can only happen when we are willing to admit change into our lives and to drop old patterns of thought and behaviour, for it was resistance to such beneficial change that caused the block in the first place, and stopped the flow of the life force that we call health.

As on the psychic plane, so on the physical plane. Physical symptoms, from a holistic point of view, are the body's attempts to right itself, to restore itself to balance. Thus it might raise body temperature to make things hot for invading bacteria, seek to throw off toxic substances by vomiting, diarrhoea or skin eruptions, make us take to our beds with some ailment or other in order to force us to rest and recharge our batteries if we are under too much stress. Being ill can fulfil our needs, and often can be the only way we can get those needs fulfilled.

At one time, I had been subjecting myself to a lot of stress, taking on more work than I could handle, overburdened with commitments that I felt obliged to keep, and wondering how on earth I was going to get the time—and the energy—to carry on at this pace. I distinctly remember thinking to myself, "I can't cope with this, it's too much," and carrying around with me the subliminal feeling that I wanted to give up, to just collapse and be looked after for a change. Soon after, I went down with the most serious illness I have had in my entire life and was admitted to hospital with a severe case of double pneumonia. Lying in that hospital bed, stoned with an escalating fever, breathing oxygen through the tube in my nose, antibiotic dripping into my arm, waking and dropping off to sleep again, I just let go of everything. That three week stay in hospital was one of the most blissful experiences of my life. Not having to *do* anything, being looked after, surrounded by concern, gentleness and caring, and, as I got better, having time to think and space to feel, with no outside expectations of me other than that I should take it easy and not exhaust myself. What a change, a 180 degree turn, from the way I had been living! It was what I really needed but had not felt able to give to myself. I had intuited it, but not acted on it. So my body had to do it for me.

"Falling ill" has its payoffs. Carl Simonton has pinpointed five of the benefits from what his patients have told him. They are:

1. Receiving permission to get out of dealing with a trouble-some problem or situation.

2. Getting attention, care, nurturing from people around them.

3. Having an opportunity to regroup their psychological energy to deal with a problem or to gain a new perspective.

4. Gaining an incentive for personal growth or for modifying undesirable habits.

5. Not having to meet their own or others' high expectations.

Simonton goes on to say, ''I believe we develop our disease for honourable reasons. It is our body's way of telling us that our needs—not just our body's needs but our emotional needs too—are not being met, and the needs that are fulfilled through our illnesses are important ones'' (*Getting Well Again*).

We participate in our illnesses more than we think. The more serious they are, the greater the changes we are being called upon to make in our lives, and especially in our ways of thinking. We create illness ourselves, albeit unconsciously, in a variety of ways to get what we need. For example, we may need the experience of being loved and cared for, or punishment for guilt. We can express our lack of self-love by not nourishing ourselves properly, as if we were not worth the trouble, by depriving ourselves of good food, rest, relaxation and enjoyable experiences. We may not speak up for ourselves and ask for what we need, as if for all the world we did not really deserve to get it. Driven by workaholism, anxiety, greed or ambition (or simply out of touch with our own rhythms and processes), unaware of our bodies beginning to groan at the stress to which we are subjecting them, we may press on, blindly hammering more nails into our own coffins. In a variety of ways we set ourselves up to be sick, not least of all by resisting change in our lives, being unwilling to discard outmoded patterns and allow new energies to come through. Fearful of the future, we cling to the past, not realising that when something has had its day it withers and dies—and can take us with it. Unaware of the damage that hanging on to old resentments is doing to our bodies in the present, we may refuse to forgive (which is not the same as to condone) and forget. Thus, albeit unwittingly, we collude with the agents of disease, the bacteria, the viruses, the carcinogens, by providing them with a fertile terrain in which to settle and thrive. In this sense, all illness can be said to be self-created.

Death

There is nothing quite like being told one has a life-threatening illness, especially if doctors think it is "incurable," for making us take stock of our lifestyles, attitudes, goals and priorities. It would appear that the patients who are willing to seek to grasp the meaning of this visitation at this particular time in their lives and to make the necessary changes stand the better chance of survival. To accept that we have somehow helped to create our own illness—even if we cannot (literally, for the life of us) figure out exactly *how*—is not at all to wallow in guilt or to beat oneself up further. The time is past for that: we have done enough of that already and in so doing have merely helped to set things up the way they are. It is time now, not for more guilt, but for more awareness, and a lot more love, above all for our suffering selves. Choosing to accept a share in responsibility for creating sickness in our bodies is in fact to move out of the position of victim, and to take back the power to heal ourselves. For what we can create, we can choose to stop creating.

A group of London researchers has found a ten year survival rate of 75% among cancer patients who reacted to diagnosis with a fighting spirit rather than with helplessness. In an article in *The Lancet* in 1975, Dr. Stephen Greer reported that the women who survive breast cancer, again, are the ones with a fighting spirit or a positive attitude. It is interesting that National Cancer Institute research psychologist Sandra Levy has found that aggressive patients tend to have more killer cells than docile patients. Patients who are considered by their physicians to be difficult or unco-operative are the ones most likely to get well. It has been said that it is the "nice" people who tend to get cancer. Perhaps it is only when confronted with the choice of survival or going under that one can give oneself permission to be more honest and to please oneself for a change, rather than living one's life as if keeping other people happy (whatever the cost to oneself) was the most important thing in the world.

Merely having surgery to remove a growth without changing the mental patterns that have manifested at a bodily level is not enough. We will merely re-create it, perhaps in another part of the body. This was the experience of Penny Brohn, co-founder of the Bristol Cancer Help Centre. She describes in her book *Gentle Giants* how she managed with the help of the Issels Clinic in Germany to pull through from breast cancer in 1979. But when, a few years later, she developed a second lump in the same breast she had to ask herself, "Why?" The answer is that the illness that developed in the body was a reflection of unresolved tensions on more subtle energy levels arising from a variety of factors, e.g., poor nutrition, stressful life-style, rigid or negative belief systems, long-held resentment or guilt, poor self-image. Unless these patterns are worked on, nothing really changes, even though the offending symptom may be physically removed, e.g., by surgery or chemotherapy. As Bernie Siegel puts it, "When a patient with a physical disease makes a thorough, positive personality change the body's defences may now eliminate the disease which is not part of the new self." *Love, Medicine and Miracles* (see Further Reading).

The more we respond with a resounding will to live, to meet the challenge, to do whatever needs to be done to restore ourselves to health, rather than with hopelessness and a "poor me" (or "why me?") response, the more likely we are to be able to pick up the pieces of our broken lives and reassemble them into a new *gestalt*, a new, healthier way of being.

Time and time again, "fatally ill" patients go into remission against the expectations of their doctors as a result of being willing to make the necessary changes in the mental patterns that have laid them low. It takes courage, honesty and guts. But, if they have the commitment and perseverence, the experience of many of them has been over and over again, that they have emerged from the crucible somehow stronger and more whole, wiser, more accepting, tolerant and loving. In retrospect, catastrophic illness can be seen to have been a blessing in disguise and a turning point in one's life.

But sometimes people find the changes that could bring healing too big to make. Perhaps they are too weak, too depressed, too identified with the old ways. At some level, they opt out, more or less consciously. We have seen that what we tell ourselves is supremely important. It can be literally a matter of life or death. And the most lethal programmes, blueprints for the body to take action on, that we can feed into our mind computer are the ones that run ''I can't cope,'' ''This is more than I can take, I want out.'' And, when we feel we've had as much as we can take, we really do opt out.

Just like illness, death can be a choice at some level, albeit a subconscious one. My mother died recently at the ripe old age of 90. She was vigorous almost to the last, or at least trying to be in spite of being crippled with arthritis and requiring regular transfusions for severe anaemia. My sister, with whom she lived, often told me how our mother would spend hours in the morning preparing for my weekly visit, putting effort into doing her hair and dressing nicely, fussing over what to prepare for our lunch together that she had been looking forward to so much all week. In spite of her weakness she put everything she had into making it just right, and with joy. By the time I turned up she would be looking good, as did the food simmering on the stove. She was a fastidious woman of the old school, of tremendous simple dignity. She was also blessed with a strong constitution that had brought her through nine pregnancies and health traumas like a hysterectomy and other surgery for cataracts and a stomach ulcer.

While I was out of the country I received a telephone call from my sister, breaking the news that my mother had had a stroke and had been taken to hospital. In response to my questioning for further details as to how she was, my sister shared with me that my mother was experiencing incontinence. Immediately, instinctively, the thought came into my mind: ''This is *It*.'' Knowing her so well, I felt that, for her, this would prove to be the last straw. And it was.

We choose to go when we no longer want to be here, when the quality of our life is such that it seems no longer worth living. The ''how'' of the exit looks after itself. Loss of the will to live is enough. In part III we will be examining the life-affirming and sustaining habits and attitudes that we should incorporate into our lives if we want to go on living, and living with quality. But first we should examine how to facilitate the healing process if we are ill by learning how to de-toxify and de-stress ourselves, by boosting our vital energy and immunity, and using the power of the mind to heal the body.

part two

HEALING

*For me, the word "incurable" simply means
that the illness cannot be cured from the
outside, but only from the inside . . .
Dissolving mental patterns dissolves disease.*

—LOUISE L. HAY

five

BEFORE WE BEGIN . . .

Physical illness is the manifestation of energy imbalance and disharmony. We have seen how, from almost imperceptible beginnings in the subtle auric layers of our energy, and tension within our consciousness this "dis-ease" within our consciousness gradually, if unchecked by prophylactic action, becomes denser and manifests as symptoms on the grosser, bodily plane. Thus, "dis-ease" becomes "disease."

Illness is a phenomenon that affects all the levels of our being. Not only do our bodies feel bad, *we* don't feel so good either, and the sort of thoughts that come into our heads as we lie on our sickbed are gloomy ones. Disease affects us physically, mentally and emotionally—and, if it is serious enough, spiritually.

Healing is the outward sign of a restoration to inner harmony and balance. Our bodies, with their marvellous built-in intelligence and survival mechanisms, will be trying instinctively to achieve this return to "law and order" from the state of "anarchy" that has been allowed to arise. It is always on our side, however it may appear. Self-healing is to consciously co-operate with this healing process ourselves, to facilitate it by removing anything that impedes it and to nourish ourselves as if we were our own sick child. We have to be our own midwives if our health is to be reborn. Gentleness is called for but also strength and commitment, and the more serious the illness, the greater the commitment needed to cure ourselves. Awareness is also needed: of what works and what doesn't in promoting recovery from illness, whatever it is, and to provide this is the intention of this second part of the book. It should be stressed again that in no way is the information given here (or indeed, anywhere else in the book) intended to *replace* treatment by a registered medical practitioner. Rather it is a sharing of how other people who are ill, often very seriously, are managing successfully to find relief—and, in many cases, remission or cure—from their ailments, and *in conjunction with regular medical care.* Your doctor should be kept informed of how you are trying to assist in your own healing process, to enhance the effectiveness of any treatment he may be giving you, and to minimise side-effects. If you are in any doubt you should ask his or her advice.

That said, however, expect professional physicians, inevitably by virtue of the nature of their medical training, to attach more weight to the purely physical means of handling illness (notably drugs), and to tend to underestimate the importance of psychological and emotional factors in healing. This is something you will have to work out between you, and you may be lucky enough to have an enlightened doctor. But whatever you do, resist any gloomy prognostications—not only from the medical profession (and, certainly if you are HIV-positive, ARC or PWA—a Person With Aids, a term invented by the media) but also from your well-meaning "realistic" friends or family. This negative input you can do without; it is un-nourishing and unproductive and can only bring you down. Rather, ask them if they love you (and, if so, to give you a hug), and tell them you love them. Remember that the agents of healing are love and *belief.* ANYTHING CAN BE HEALED. So, be realistic, PLAN FOR A MIRACLE.

Some of the suggestions given in this section will be primarily aimed at healing through the body, others through the mind or the emotions. Always remember, however, that these distinctions are in fact purely arbitrary and not isolated "bits" of us. Whatever we do in the one area will resonate in the others. We are always trying to heal the WHOLE, and, indeed, "healing" means a "making whole."

For convenience we shall be considering the factors that

have been shown over and over again to facilitate getting well again, often against all expectations. They are as follows. Think of them as the Ten Commandments of Healing:

> DE-STRESS YOURSELF
> DETOXIFY YOUR BODY
> NOURISH YOUR IMMUNE SYSTEM
> BOOST YOUR VITALITY
> LET GO OF ALL NEGATIVITY
> AFFIRM THE POSITIVE
> VISUALISE HEALTH
> LOVE YOURSELF MORE—AND MORE
> EXPRESS YOUR FEELINGS
> LISTEN TO YOUR INNER SELF

We have to work on our energy system from two directions: on strengthening our weakened body and repairing and stimulating its own defence mechanisms; and on clearing, balancing and restoring the flow of energy on the more subtle mental, emotional and spiritual planes, where in fact the roots of our illness are to be found. In each area we shall be calling on the power of the mind to heal through affirmations and visualisations.

Healing oneself is a very individual process. Its essence is getting back in touch, in tune, with oneself and contacting the healer within—our innate wisdom that always knows what is right for us. Treat what follows, therefore, as suggestions for you to work with as and when they feel right, rather than things you have to do, and all at once. They are there for your support—a compendium of what others have found and are finding helps them to feel better and, in many cases, to get better.

six

DE-STRESSING YOURSELF

The latest evidence of research, as we saw in Part I, seems to be bearing out that the biggest single reason why we fall ill is exposure to too much or too prolonged stress. Unless we actually enjoy it as a challenge, stress depresses and affects our immune system, our energy levels, our state of mind and the quality of our lives. It therefore makes sense to make de-stressing ourselves a top priority when we are ill. The body will want to do this instinctively in any way it can. We will feel like lying down and sleeping a lot, withdrawing from work commitments or cancelling social engagements, just as a sick pet will be lethargic and "switched off" and disappear into some remote corner of the house where it can rest undisturbed. This "switching off" from involvement in activity in the outside world is the essence of the de-stressing process, for it was "overdoing it" and over-exposure to stress that probably helped to bring us down in the first place.

"First Aid" for Stress

The "first aid" for stress is to withdraw from unnecessary activity of body and mind in order to recharge our batteries. It is a decision to let go of all "shoulds" arising from others' expectations (or our own expectations of ourselves) and to choose to put ourselves and our needs FIRST. Particularly, we need to give ourselves time and space in which to handle the trauma our systems are undergoing.

The rest of this chapter deals with things which will help us achieve this.

BACH "RESCUE REMEDY" (NUMBER 39)

The 39 Bach Remedies are prepared from the flowers of wild plants, bushes, and trees, and are useful for treating a wide range of sources of emotional tension. None of them is harmful or habit-forming. Their discoverer, Dr. Edward Bach, became convinced that all illness was the result of underlying negative mental states. He gave up his lucrative Harley Street practice in 1930 to devote his whole time to seeking energies in the plant world which would restore vitality to the sick by correcting these negative states (such as worry, hopelessness, irritability, etc). The 39 remedies cover every known negative state of mind.

The "Rescue Remedy" is a combination of five other Bach remedies: (Cherry Plum; Clematis; Impatiens; Rock Rose and Star of Bethlehem) and is an all-purpose emergency composite for shock, terror, panic, emotional upsets, etc. It is especially indicated if the onset of the indisposition has been particularly upsetting, for example, following the shock of bad news, the result of an accident, or heralded by a panic-producing medical diagnosis.

The Rescue Remedy really does work—and fast—to soothe jangled nerves. On the morning of my mother's funeral the family had left to me the job of opening the front door for the mourners who were gathering at my sister's house before the arrival of the hearse and the cars which were to take us to the cemetery. Each time I answered the doorbell and was met by a face that clearly showed that the owner was very distressed and was having a hard job handling it on this formal occasion (mostly, it turned out, my nieces and nephews, who had adored their grandmother), I led them off to the kitchen first for a "nip" of Bach Rescue Remedy. They all drank it obediently, too choked and dazed even to ask what it was. It did not suppress the grief they were feeling, but they now felt less overwhelmed by it and less afraid of cracking up.

We shall be listing all the Bach Flower Remedies in another section (see page 109) when we come to consider ways of antidoting the negative mental states that, it has been suggested, are any underlying cause of illness, and indicating where to get hold of them.

SLEEP

Sleep is the "great restorer." It is Nature's way of reducing our energy output to the minimum so that our batteries can be recharged and energy can be directed to the parts of the body in the "front line" for healing.

Sleep as much as you need to—and whenever you feel like dozing off. Getting well again is very much about getting back into tune with your own bodily rhythms, respecting your needs from moment to moment—and asking for what you need. So, for example, if your hospital bed is surrounded by visitors and you are starting to feel drained, give yourself permission to tell them that you need to take a nap. Being in a crisis situation is not the time for being over-polite. And, if your visitors are sensitive, love you and want you to get well, they will understand and not be offended.

DEEP RELAXATION SESSIONS

Sometimes you may not be able to sleep, or, in the periods when you are awake, may be tense (perhaps because of pain) or anxious about your condition. Gloomy thoughts that refuse to go away can drain us just as much as the stressful outside situations from which we may have withdrawn physically. The stress is now inside our heads. And that means tension in our bodies, for anxious thoughts give rise to disturbing feelings which make us tense our muscles for "fight or flight."

Relaxing as deeply as we can, as often as we can, brings many benefits to health. We recharge our batteries with vital energy, take the strain off our muscles and internal organs, strengthen our immune system, and therefore feel better and look better. We resurface from a session of deep relaxation feeling more at peace, more optimistic, and refreshed.

This is because of the physiological changes that take place when our brain wavelength frequency drops from Beta to Alpha. Respiration slows down and the heart rate decreases by an average of three beats a minute. There is a decrease in the level of blood lactate, associated with anxiety states. Blood pressure also drops, as does oxygen consumption and more so than in sleep. What is happening is that as the sympathetic nervous system goes into abeyance and the parasympathetic nervous system takes over, a decrease in the rate of the body's metabolism takes place. What this means is that being in Alpha causes our energy resources to be taxed less, which is obviously especially desirable when we are ill. Apart from sleep (and hibernation), sinking into the Alpha state is the *only* way to achieve this deeply restful hypo-metabolism. Just to lie quietly is not enough, especially if our minds are still racing with thoughts. By *deep* relaxation we mean *total* relaxation of body, mind and emotions. Resting and revitalising ourselves in this Alpha state is the biggest single antidote to stress there is, and very healing at all levels.

How then do we achieve it? Practise the Alpha Plan for Total Relaxation described below at least once a day, and, even better, preferably two or three times daily. After meals is a particularly good time, for your energy will be naturally moving down into your body for handling digestion so as a result you will tend to feel more lethargic than at other times.

The Alpha Plan is based both on the experience and practice of eastern meditators and yogis who charted the pathways to the Alpha state in their quest for enlightenment, and on the research of modern medical scientists interested in finding methods that work to combat the growing toll from stress disease. If you are interested in knowing more about these and on what the Alpha Plan is based you can read about it in detail in my book *Total Relaxation in Five Steps—The Alpha Plan* (Penguin 1989).

THE ALPHA PLAN FOR TOTAL RELAXATION

Stage 1: "Senses Relaxed"

1. Take a few slow, deep breaths.

2. Become aware of tension around the eyes. Unfocus them (eyes closed) until they feel very "soft."

3. Listen passively to sounds from the outside that are reaching you. Just allow them to be there, without trying to identify them. After a few minutes of this "tuning in" move on to the next stage.

Stage 2: "Feelings Positive"

Repeat several times, silently and slowly, a phrase or sentence which cancels out any upsetting thoughts or panic you may be experiencing. You could use the favourite "all-rounder" of Emile Coué, the founder of auto-suggestion: "Every day, in every way, I am getting better and better."

In the section later in Part II entitled "Affirm the Positive" you will find others you might like to use as being more "on target," more specifically geared to, for example, worry about your health.

Stage 3: "Mind Slowing Down"

1. Become aware of your breathing. Without changing it in any way, simply start to count after each exhalation. "One" . . . (breathe in . . . breathe out . . .) "Two" . . . (breathe in . . . breathe out . . .) "Three" . . . and so on up to "Ten," and then start another round with "One" . . .

2. After a few rounds of counting in this way, substitute a word that has calming associations for you instead of the number. Any word that does not have disturbing associations for you and that suggests feeling peaceful, calm or safe will do. Try, for example, repeating between the out-breath and the inbreath one of the following:

> *Relax* or *Relaxing*
> *Peace* or *Peaceful*
> *Love*
> *Bliss* or *Blissful*

After a few rounds of repeating your mantra (for this is what the word is) your mind will have slowed down sufficiently for you to begin to be more aware of what you are experiencing in the way of body sensations. By deliberately feeding more attention to these body sensations we move into deeper body awareness—which is the same as relaxation.

Stage 4: "Body Relaxing"

In this stage, then, we progressively relax the whole body, simply by trying to become more aware, in turn, of the different parts of it, starting with the feet and ending up with the face and scalp. We try to *feel* each part in turn, allowing ourselves to feel first how much tension there is in this part of the body, and then letting go of it.

Start with the big toe of the left foot. Without twiddling it, let your attention feel it from the inside, its size and shape . . . From there, after ten seconds or so, let your attention roam over the toes of the left foot in turn (once again without twiddling them), just being as aware of them as you can, one after the other.

Now feel the rest of the left foot; your heel resting on the mattress . . . the sole, so sensitive to tickling . . . the hard bones on the top of the instep . . . *Take your time.*

Now feel the weight of the whole left foot . . . Feel it being supported by the mattress and imagine it getting heavier and heavier, sinking into the mattress . . . And let go of it.

Move on now to the left ankle. Feel "from the inside" its shape . . . the hardness of the bones . . . Move upwards to the calf muscle and feel whether it is tense or relaxed . . . Imagine it expanding, loosening, getting softer . . . Become aware of your shin bone, the hardness of it . . . Remember how painful it feels when you bang it on something . . . Feel your left knee-

cap . . . What shape is it, how big? . . . From the kneecap progress to the left thigh . . . How tense is the big muscle at the
front? Feel the tension—and let go of it . . . Try to feel the
length and size of the left thighbone . . .

Now let your awareness scan the whole of the left leg that
you have just relaxed . . . Relax it even more by imagining it
getting heavier and heavier, sinking into the mattress . . . Notice how much heavier it feels than the right, unrelaxed leg
. . . And let go of it.

Repeat the same sequence with the right foot and leg, once
again starting at the toes.

When both legs are totally relaxed, allow yourself to become aware in turn of the other parts of your body. Spend as
much time as you need relaxing each part before moving on.
With each part:

a) feel it first "from the inside," its size and shape

b) feel how relaxed or how tense it is—and "relax into the
tension"

c) imagine that part getting heavier, softer, loosening up . . .

d) let go of it.

Scan the whole body in the following sequence:

> buttocks
> anus and genitals
> lower back
> spine
> shoulders
> left arm (upper, elbow, forearm, wrist)
> left hand (palm, back of hand, thumb, fingers in turn)
> right arm (upper, elbow, forearm, wrist)
> right hand (palm, back of hand, thumb, fingers in turn)
> belly (imagine that this part is expanding, opening up)
> chest (breathe slow and deep into the heart area . . . Give
> a few deep sighs, imagining as you do so that you are
> cleansing and energising your heart) . . .

- Feel the whole weight of your torso . . . Let it get heavier, expand, sink down . . .

- Feel the tension that comes from "having to face the world"—in your jaw, mouth, tongue . . . Let your face sag, and your jaw drop . . . Feel the tension around the eyes . . . Let your eyes become soft . . . Feel as if they are sinking deep into their sockets . . .

- End with the scalp. Feel any tightness, and wiggle your ears to relax it . . . Remember how nice it feels when your hairdresser is shampooing your hair, how soothing to have your scalp massaged under a jet of warm water . . .

Stage 5: "Letting Go"

By now you should be in a totally passive, totally relaxed state, very much in your body rather than in your head and feeling calm and peaceful. Deepen this state by continuing to feed attention to whatever you are aware of in your body for, remember, body awareness *is* relaxation. Just let go . . . and enjoy the blissful Alpha state for as long as you want. You deserve it.

Summary of the Stages of the Alpha Plan

Stage 1:

Eyes closed, unfocussed, "soft," "just listening" (relaxes the senses).

Stage 2:

Repetition of a reassuring phrase (relaxes emotional tension).

Stage 3:

Counting the breaths and repeating your calming mantra (relaxes the mind).

Stage 4:

Body scanning (relaxes the muscles and internal organs).

Stage 5:

Body awareness/resting in Alpha (letting go of all tension).

When you decide to come out of your deep relaxation session, do so gradually, to avoid the jarring effect of shooting straight up from Alpha into Beta again. (This is what happens, for example, if the alarm clock on a normal working-day doesn't go off and we wake up, look at it, probably curse it—and have to rush out of bed, and out of the house without breakfast.) This applies not only after finishing a deep relaxation session but also after doing any of the visualisations we shall be suggesting in this book.

To avoid feeling disorientated therefore, give yourself a few minutes to ground yourself by:

a) tuning in to the sounds you can hear

b) taking a few deep breaths

c) stretching and relaxing your body

d) opening your eyes, looking around the room and reminding yourself where you are.

RELAXING VISUALISATIONS

When you are totally relaxed, in the final, "let-go" stage of the Alpha Plan, you will find that this is the best time to practise the visualisations to be described throughout the book and, of course, any others you choose to dream up for yourself. Below I give you two visualisations to enjoy which will also help the "relaxation response." Once you get the hang of visualising you can make up your own. Any scene you choose to create in your mind will do, so long as it makes you feel safe and you enjoy it.

Beach Visualisation

Imagine the most inviting beach you can think of. It could be one that you have already known and enjoyed, perhaps on holiday—or it could be your own idea of what a perfect beach should look like. See in your mind's eye all the features that make it so inviting. Make your visualisation as detailed and as vivid as possible.

For example, is the sea a clear; limpid blue-green, calm and gently lapping the sand? Or is it in wilder mood, with white crested waves crashing on to the beach and foaming back again with a hiss?

See the colour of the sand (or is it a pebble beach?) and how far the beach extends in each direction, possibly with palm trees, or fringed with oleander or bougainvillea. (If you want them there, put them there!) Look out to sea. Can you see boats or distant sails, or is it clear to the horizon?

Feel yourself there, part of this sundrenched scene. How are you enjoying yourself? Swimming, perhaps, or just floating lazily on your back, eyes closed against the bright sunshine warming your face while seabirds cry and wheel overhead in the bluest of skies . . .

Perhaps you are lying in the surf, allowing the waves to break and swirl over and around you, enjoying the ebb and flow and the coolness of the water on your body . . .

See yourself later relaxing full-length on your gaily-coloured towel or your air-bed, luxuriating in the warmth of the sun, feeling all the tension in your body evaporating with the drops of water upon it . . .

Are you alone with your drowsy thoughts or have you brought a companion with you? If so, turn over and enjoy the sensual experience of having your back and legs massaged gently with suntan oil. Smell its fragrance as you just surrender to the caring attention of this person whom you trust and with whom you feel totally at ease . . .

Garden Visualisation

Visualise the most beautiful garden you have ever been in—or create your own ideal garden.

See yourself in this garden, perhaps strolling across a beautifully trimmed lawn that is fringed by flowering shrubs and neatly laid-out flower beds. Stop to admire the colours of the azaleas and rhododendrons, to sniff the fragrance of this rose . . . Hear the buzz of the insects (or perhaps the faint drone of a jet high overhead), sounds that seem only to heighten the sense of peace, of being at one with Nature that you feel . . .

Once again, make your visualisation as detailed and as enjoyable for yourself as you can. (One of the advantages of visualising over real life is that money is no object—and everything is possible!) Treat yourself, for example, to a couple of peacocks strutting on the lawn, one perhaps proudly displaying the gorgeous, shimmering blue-green tail feathers, wheeling gently to impress . . . And perhaps a fishpond with waterlilies, under whose flat leaves you catch the odd flash of golden orange of its inhabitants . . .

The most important thing to remember when doing a visualisation is to include yourself in the video you are running and to get the feeling in your body that it is all actually happening.

Music

To make your deep relaxation sessions and visualisations even more enjoyable you might like to play taped music while you work through them. If you are in hospital you can do this on a Walkman to avoid disturbing any other patients who may be in the room.

Quite apart from simply providing a pleasant background, music *per se* has healing properties. When we listen to soothing music we enjoy, relaxing physiological changes take place in our bodies. Listening to music has exactly the opposite effect to anger on the body; it lowers blood pressure, slows down the pulse rate, aids the digestive process by restoring the flow of gastric juices to the stomach, and has an overall relaxing effect upon the body.

Pythagoras was a firm believer in the therapeutic power of music for both mind and body and included it in the curriculum for his students at his academy at Crotona.

Subjectively, music can be soothing and calming, and also
moving and inspirational, for it gets us in the heart chakra and
stimulates the right (the intuitive/feeling) side of the brain. It
has been found by psychiatrists that music is a great mood
changer and can help us shift quickly out of depression, hopelessness, grief and despair.

Appropriately selected music, therefore, can enhance the
depth of your relaxation, and also facilitate the focussing on
positive, calming images when visualising. Experiments have
shown that, for the purposes of healing and relaxation, instrumental is better than vocal music. It should be slow rather
than fast (the last thing you want is to get your feet tapping
under the sheets, at least, not while you're trying to relax!) It
should be soft, rather than loud—just providing a background
to your descent into Alpha or your visualisation.

There is a type of instrumental music called "New Age"
which is particularly suitable for using as a background to
deep relaxation, visualisation or meditation (which we shall be
discussing later). You may well already be familiar with, say,
the work of Kitaro, or Deuter. If you are not, the (far from
elegant) words that come to mind to convey the atmosphere
created by such music would be something like "floaty,"
"flowing" and "spacy." New Age composers use synthesis-
ers, chimes, flutes, harps—all basically "gentle" instruments—
which, if I may be allowed to mis-quote, really do have
charms to "soothe the savage beast" of tension and stress.

If you like classical music, remember that experiments have
proved that baroque music is the most effective for promoting
the "relaxation response," probably because of its ordered
structure and recurring melodic and harmonic sequences that
suggest clear boundaries and therefore make us feel safe.

Some suggestions for tapes of relaxing music you might like
to try out for yourself are listed in the Appendix (see pages
193–7). Also well worth investing in are tapes of "environmental sounds," for example, the sound of running water
(surely one of the most soothing sounds of all), ocean waves
ebbing and flowing, or sweet birdsong.

Give Yourself More Time, More Space

Be quite ruthless with this. When you are ill it must be your
top priority not to allow yourself to be stressed by anyone or
anything if you are to get well again. Don't do anything you
don't feel like doing, don't allow visits from people who are
likely, from past experience, to drain you. You have the best
excuse in the world, perhaps for the first time in your life, for
choosing not to meet outside expectations for a while; you are
not well. Make the most of it while it lasts. And be particularly
ruthless with the workaholic inside you, the part of you that
is likely to fret at all the things that are piling up and may try
to make you feel guilty at just taking it easy for a change.
This may well be the subpersonality within you that has been
most responsible for laying you low in the first place, by making you "overdo it" and take on more work than you can
cope with.

Enjoy as Much as You Can

Remember Norman Cousins and the healing power of laughter. The Marx Brothers may not be your cup of tea, and you
may loathe *Candid Camera*. So find other things to enjoy.
These could be music, reading, or television (especially the
nonviolent, more nourishing programmes such as comedies or
films about love and Nature that remind you how beautiful
people, animals and this planet of ours really are).

Remember how what you choose to look at affects your
body and particularly your immune system, so expose yourself
to as little negative input as possible. And if you don't have
anything to laugh at, laugh anyway—to yourself. It may seem
false at first, but it does get funnier as you get into it. Exercise
those laughter muscles and know that you are doing yourself
a whole power of good.

Have the intention to enjoy yourself in spite of your illness,
rather than brooding over it and bringing yourself down with
worry. What we tell ourselves is supremely important. On
awakening in the morning decide that you will find things to
enjoy today, and such is the nature of our mind-computers that
you will. You will be "set" to notice only the positive, and

the people you come in contact with will resonate with this and lighten up when they are with you. The negative, of course, will still be there but you won't notice it. You will attract the sort of experiences that go with your positive self-programming, some of them, perhaps, pleasant surprises: a visit from a friend you haven't seen in a long while maybe, a letter full of loving energy wishing you a speedy recovery, flowers and (on a particularly good day!) presents.

Try to stay positive, for your own sake, for life gives you more of where you are at already. The more positive you are the better you will feel.

Handling Pain

"Easier said than done," you may be thinking, especially if you are experiencing pain or discomfort in your body. And yet a large part of the experience of pain is to do with tension. We contract our muscles against it, we worry about what it means, we fear that it may get worse. Thus, as well as having a pain, we torture ourselves further—and make it worse.

Assuming that your doctor has already treated the source of the pain with appropriate medication and has done all he can do, the only thing *you* can do is to try to relax as deeply as you can in some of the following ways:

• *Breathe into the pain.* Imagine you are sending healing, soothing energy to the part that is inflamed or hurting—and you will be, for energy follows thought.

• *Talk to the pain.* Ask it for information about itself. Why is it there, for example? What is its message for you? Ask it what you could do to make it feel better. And listen for answers. Pain is always a *message*. In a later section we shall be discussing in more detail the importance of listening to what the body is trying to tell us, why we got ill in the first place and what we need to do to get better.

• *Try to feel the pain MORE.* It sounds paradoxical, but in so doing you will take the "edge" off it. This is because, by engaging it, "going to meet it," instead of shrinking away from it, you will stop contracting and holding muscles and relax into it. Try to *see* the pain in your mind's eye. What area—exactly—does the pain cover? What *colour* is it? What *shape* is it? The images that will come to mind will probably be fluctuating ones. As you watch, the pain will change size, shape and colour. Stay with these images. Keep watching and feeling it. As you pursue it in this way with your attention it will probably start to get smaller, fainter in outline and colour, less virulent . . . With a bit of luck it may even disappear entirely (this is often particularly the case with headaches caused by tension) but at least you will find it easier to put up with.

Now would be a good time to relax even further by "going down to Alpha" and/or listening to music you love or soothing environmental sounds.

Possibly because of its ability to make us relax, music has come to be regarded over the last 30 years as a valuable therapeutic tool. It has been used successfully at a Montreal hospital as a painkiller, for example, and for facilitating easy childbirth at the Medical Center of the University of Kansas. There it was found that playing background music in the delivery room made labours easier—and less pain-killing drugs had to be used. In Poland a study of over 400 people suffering from severe headaches and different types of neurological illness revealed that those who listened regularly to music were able, after six months, to do without most of their drugs. A control group who did not listen to music still needed to take the full dose of painkillers to secure relief.

Ask for Support

Ask for any sort of help you feel you need, and from anyone you can trust to give it. It could be help of a very practical kind, if you are house-bound, like asking someone to collect your prescription for you or your pension from the Post Office, to shop for food or, if you are too weak to do it yourself, getting someone to write a letter claiming sickness benefit for you. Or it could be emotional support you need—and the importance of this for healing cannot be too highly emphasised, especially in those moments (usually at night) when you start to get the "blues" or to experience panic. I attribute my full recovery from double pneumonia in a Copenhagen hospital partly to superb medical attention (Denmark's Health Service must surely be one of the finest in the world). But also to the kindness and patience of the nursing staff who would come in every hour during the night to take my temperature and, sensing how I felt—weak as a kitten, a little lost and a long way from home—were willing just to sit on the bed and hold my hand, to reassure and simply be there for me. It made a difference.

But you may have to ask for it. Don't assume that everybody knows what's going on with you, especially if you are accustomed to putting on a brave face. Healing yourself is also about being honest and upfront with your true feelings. *The American Journal of Medical Science* reported in 1977 that of 120 patients who had had a mastectomy the preceding year, in each case interpersonal support had contributed substantially to their coping with post-mastectomy depression. So, if you are fortunate enough to be living with someone you love, when you are not feeling so good, when the child inside you is feeling vulnerable and scared, share this with them—and ask for a hug, to be held. Support does not always have to be given in words.

seven

DETOXIFYING YOUR BODY

In hatha yoga ill health is thought to be the result of a lack of vital energy (*prana*) together with intoxication of the bowel. As a result, a healthy diet and inner cleansing practices form a large part of the traditional discipline of the yogi, as well as the better known breathing exercises (*pranayama*) and postures (*asanas*) designed to strengthen the vital force.

It has been suggested that in fact the presence of germs in a sick person is not so much the *cause* of disease but the *result* of a toxic system. In other words, these micro-organisms gather to feed off a toxic body in rather the same way as worms and flies congregate around putrid meat. Whether this is true or not, certainly the more toxins we have in our bodies the less healthy we shall be or feel. Just remember how you feel after too much alcohol, cigarettes, sweets or junk food, or, even worse, if you are unlucky enough to come down with a case of food-poisoning. The body literally gets ''sick and tired'' of toxins.

GOOD AND BAD FOODS

Most of us probably now take the trouble to scrutinise the labels on the supermarket tins and packets for the content of additives, denoted by the letter ''E'': colourings, preservatives, antioxydants, emulsifiers and stabilisers. Many more people today are vegetarian, non-smokers, and concerned about environmental pollution and carcinogens. But many of us, too, are still addicted to meat, sugar, coffee, alcohol, and perhaps even tranquillisers. With luck, or a strong constitution, we may get away with it.

But if we do get ill, our symptoms are often our body's attempts to throw out the junk we have been putting into it: nausea, diarrhoea, fever, skin rashes, boils and abscesses, bronchitis and so forth. In homoeopathy it is through the skin and the lungs that the body may start to discharge toxins if a remedy is working. These toxins can also put a strain on the liver and kidneys, and indeed on other organs, including the heart. In other words, eliminating toxins puts the body under stress. In this section we examine how we can help ourselves to get better if we are ill by co-operating with our body's attempts to ''clean up our act,'' rather than sabotaging the process by putting more rubbish into it.

Avoid, or at Least Cut Down On . . .

Alcohol

Really, alcohol is not a stimulant at all, but depresses all the cells of our body. However we usually refer to it as a stimulant, because it lessens brain activity and thus deadens anxiety.

Alcohol is fermented sugar. It makes hard work for the liver and is consumed at the expense of vitamin B6 which, we shall be seeing in the next section, is a crucial nutrient of the immune system.

For about 60 years alcohol has been found to be associated with increased risk of cancer, particularly of the gastrointestinal and upper respiratory tracts—though why this should be so is not clear, since it does not produce cancer in laboratory animals. In 1983 Sandler named it as an immunosuppressant and it may stimulate the production of free radicals (molecular fragments capable of damaging cells, producing genetic damage and perhaps even causing cancer).

Yet, on the other hand, it must be said that treating oneself to one or two glasses of wine a day has actually been shown to protect against coronary heart disease. Surveys have also suggested that people who indulge in small amounts of alcohol tend to live longer and suffer fewer illnesses than teetotallers.

It seems that we have to recognise the stress-relieving properties of the odd drink and be sensible and non-rigid about it. This, at any rate, is the appproach at the Bristol Cancer Help Centre, where doctors and nutritionists allow patients to enjoy the odd drink, largely because of co-founder Penny Brohn's experience at the Issels Clinic where she was advised to do likewise. One scientific study actually suggested that a good boost for the immune system would be a combination of small amounts of alcohol plus vitamin C and oil of evening primrose.

Therefore, if you fancy a glass of wine or a beer, the odd one probably won't do you any harm. The relaxing effect of moderate drinking must be balanced against the alcohol's toxicity. And it's up to each individual to decide what "moderate" means. Certainly some might consider the British Medical Association's guideline of 1 litre of wine, 2 pints of beer, or 7 ounces of alcohol in any 24 hour period rather excessive!

What you must definitely avoid is going on a binge, and especially so if you are being treated with drugs. Cancer patients, for example, will already have their livers working overtime to detoxify the by-products of cancer cells and the effects of drugs. And abuse of alcohol can lead to deficiencies in nutrients that play a role in immune functioning.

Caffeine

Caffeine is found not only in coffee, but also in black tea (i.e., tea brewed from black as opposed to green tea leaves), cocoa and cola drinks. Caffeine has been suspected of contributing to cancer (especially of the pancreas, the fourth most common cause of cancer deaths) and heart disease. It is rather like adrenalin in its stimulation of the nervous system and the heart and the dilation of blood vessels. Just drinking small amounts of coffee increases by ten times the formation in the stomach of nitrosamines, some of which are known to be carcinogens.

It would seem that, if you really must have your coffee, you should not have more than three cups per day, for the risk goes up after that. And avoid artificial sweeteners or drinking out of plastic or foam cups for these have been suspected of being implicated in the ''cancer connection'' of coffee.

Sugar

Give sugar up entirely, for it is absolutely no good for you. It is the junkiest of junk foods, with absolutely no nutritional value. In order to digest it we plough into our precious reserves of vitamin B, stress our digestive systems, and make the liver and pancreas work overtime to produce glycogen and insulin to try to compensate and keep our blood sugar at an acceptable level. Sugar *leeches* vitamins, minerals and energy from our bodies. This, especially when we are ill, we can do without.

Taking sugar in tea or coffee accounts for about 50% of the average person's consumption of sugar which is about 110 lbs. a year. But remember that sugar is added to a wide range of supermarket items, like soft drinks, canned fruits, certain kinds of pickles, and even some packet soups. And next time you reach for that slice of chocolate cake, remember that it probably contains the equivalent of ten and a half teaspoons of sugar . . .

Meat

Many people today have stopped eating meat, or are cutting down on it, for the following health reasons:

1. Animal fat, which meat is rich in, is conducive to heart disease—the world's biggest killer today.

2. Meat is hard to digest and causes putrefaction in the bowel. Toxins are absorbed via the colon and this could possibly contribute to bowel cancer, the second commonest form of cancer in Britain.

3. Flesh foods contain sodium salts which tend to make the blood acid. A slightly alkaline blood stream is needed for good health.

4. The blood of slaughtered animals often contains antibiotics and other drugs which have been administered to prevent or combat disease.

5. On their way to being slaughtered the animals will probably have in their panic produced adrenalin which we then ingest, to the detriment of our immune systems.

The consumption of red meat should be cut down and eventually eliminated if we are ill. Chicken, too, has its risks, notably the antibiotics administered to battery hens to counteract disease caused by overcrowding and the danger of salmonella, especially if the bird is under-cooked. Substitute fish—it's better for you, especially fish from the open oceans, as inland waters may be polluted and affect the quality of the flesh.

Other Things to Avoid . . .

ice-cream

pasteurised cheeses

fried food

white flour products

roasted and/or salted nuts (especially peanuts)

refined fats and oils (unsaturated as well as saturated)

salt

pepper

anything containing "E" numbers or artificial additives

anything with food additives (e.g., monosodium glutamate), artificial flavours, preservatives and colours.

In addition, any foods high in cholesterol are to be avoided. High fat diets not only are conducive to heart disease but also impair immune functioning. This includes ice-cream and fried foods (which are also hard to digest). Ice-cream also often contains additives (e.g., artificial flavourings).

Foods made with white flour are not nutritious because the vitamin-bearing husk of the grain has been removed. They provide few nutrients and many calories. On the other hand, whole (unpolished grains) are not only nutritious, but also provide fibre for a healthy colon and regular elimination (see below).

Good for Detoxifying

Fibre

Fibre speeds up the passage of waste matter through the bowel and therefore the rapid disposal of toxins from the colon. Cereal bran is the best known form, but we get fibre also from fruit and vegetables. We should consume about 1 oz of fibre each day (25–30 gms). The table opposite will give you some idea of where exactly you can get fibre from, and also how much.

Nuts also have a high fibre content (especially almonds, brazil nuts, hazelnuts, coconuts, peanuts and walnuts), as are blackberries, loganberries and raspberries.

Brown Rice

Brown rice is also rich in fibre. When eaten with lightly-cooked or steamed vegetables and/or pulses it is considered by followers of a macrobiotic diet to be just about the healthiest and most balanced meal we human beings can eat. As well as helping detoxification, it is easy on the digestion and very nourishing and therefore a desirable thing to eat regularly when we are ill, especially if we have been recently eating a lot of junk food.

In case you have not tried cooking brown rice before, here's how to do it. Heat a *little* vegetable oil (preferably virgin olive oil or grape-seed oil) in a saucepan and stir in 1 cup of rice when the oil is hot. When the rice grains are coated with the oil, add 2½ cups of cold water. Cover the saucepan with a

Cereals	Quantity	Dietary fibre in grams
Unprocessed bran	2 tablespoons	9
Bran breakfast cereal	6 "	8
Wheat breakfast cereal	2 pieces	6
Cornflakes	3 spoons	1
Porridge	6 spoons	2
Wholemeal bread	1 slice	4
Vegetables		
Baked beans	4 tablespoonfuls	7
Sweetcorn	3 "	3
Lentils	2 tablespoonfuls	3
Cauliflower	1 medium portion	2
Potatoes	"	2
Lettuce	6 leaves	1
Fruits		
Banana	1 medium size	4
Orange	"	2
Apple	"	2
Pineapple	1 thick slice	2

lid, bring the water to the boil, then turn the heat right down and allow to simmer until most of the liquid has been absorbed. Test the rice for chewiness. If the texture is to your taste, remove the lid and allow the rest of the water to evaporate. If it is still too chewy, add a *little* more water and continue to cook.

Raw Vegetables and Fruits

These, as well as being fibre-rich, are also "living" foods and therefore will not putrefy in the bowel. The best time to eat raw foods is for lunch, so you give yourself plenty of time to digest them (though fruit for breakfast with muesli or bran makes a good start to the day). You will find plenty of ideas for delicious recipes in Leslie Kenton's classic *Raw Energy*, listed under Further Reading at the back of this book (see page 191). How much raw food to include in your diet depends on the state of your digestion, but try to aim for at least 25% of your daily intake.

Fruit and Vegetable Juices and Herb Teas

It is important to drink a lot of fluid (at least 3 litres a day), and especially when you are ill. Some hospitals in fact make the patient record every time he or she has something to drink in order to keep a check that adequate intake of fluids is happening. Since stimulating drinks are not advisable, most of this intake should be in the form of water (preferably mineral water), fruit juices (preferably freshly-squeezed, or at least not of the "long-life" variety) and herb teas. Raw juices have no equal for keeping an alkaline balance of the blood. Carrot juice is particularly detoxifying since it contains so much Beta-Carotene (vitamin A). Rosehip tea is very high on vitamin C content, and camomile and fresh mint teas are particularly cleansing. Freshly-squeezed lemon juice flavoured with pure honey is also purifying, especially if taken first thing in the morning with a spoonful of cider vinegar.

Vitamin C

We shall be discussing the immune-enhancing power of this vitamin in the next section. Suffice to say here that in its role as an antioxydant and free radical scavenger, vitamin C is a powerful detoxifier and helps to prevent the formation of carcinogens in the body. Since we cannot store this vitamin we need a fresh supply every day—and especially if we are on aspirin, antibiotics, or if we smoke. (We lose 25mg of vitamin C with each cigarette). We shall also be discussing later how much of this vitamin to take and in what form to take it, since there has been some controversy in this area.

Garlic

The purifying properties of garlic have been known from time immemorial, but it is only recently that we have realised its power as an anti-viral agent. It is particularly good for cleansing the digestive system, also (like onions) for helping to clear mucus from the respiratory system. It has even been claimed that garlic has worked where some antibiotics have failed to clear up bacterial infections. So take garlic daily when you are ill, raw in salads, for example, or cooked in sauces. To get rid of the smell you can chew fresh parsley as well—or take garlic oil in capsules instead of the raw cloves.

Lactobacillus Acidophilus

This is useful to take whenever you are on a course of antibiotics (or, indeed, other drugs) to replace beneficial bacteria in the gut and aid digestion. A disturbed flora in the gastrointestinal tract (caused by such drugs) can set up an environment favourable to yeast proliferation, for example *Candida albicans*. Acidophilus is present in live yoghurts, or it can be bought separately.

CLEANSING AFFIRMATIONS AND VISUALISATIONS

How one eats is almost as important as what one eats. Foods will nourish us better if we are in a calm state of mind at mealtimes and give attention to really tasting what we are putting into our mouths, rather than, say, watching television or reading a newspaper while we do so. Food should be really *chewed*, or as they say in yoga, "Drink your food and eat your drinks."

The time-honoured religious custom of saying grace before (and giving thanks after) meals made nutritional sense. It forced us to be aware of what we were putting into our mouths—and relaxed us at the same time. Not only that, but it harmonised the foodstuff's vibrations with our own. If that sounds a little crazy, remember that everything has its own type of vibrations, its own aura (which, as we have seen can actually be photographed). It would seem that all matter has some degree of consciousness, however little. Physicists have proved that matter is affected by the observer: we affect in a subtle but measurable way everything we look at. Attention is energy, so whatever we give our attention to we energise. How

much more will we affect things if we actually *talk* to them . . .
Certainly we know this is so in the case of plants and may well
be so in the case of more inanimate matter. So before you eat
and drink, bless your food, believe it will do you good and it
will.

Similarly, instead of absent-mindedly popping your pills (or
even worse, thinking how unpleasant they taste and how you
would rather not have to be taking them at all), give yourself
a moment to become aware of why you are taking them at all,
to help your body cope with whatever it is going through.
Think of these drugs as friends, and even if it does feel a bit
silly, talk to them as such. At the very least you will be programming your body to receive them without resistance—
which means side-effects.

I have a client with AIDS who comes for counselling. He
hates drugs of any kind and would never even take an aspirin
for a headache. To his dismay his physicians at the hospital
put him on a regime of AZT (Retrovir)—no less than 12 tablets to be taken at intervals throughout the day, the last four
at night before going to bed. At first he refused, but the doctors
convinced him that, with his severely damaged immune system, his only defence against the HIV virus was to take them.
They explained how AZT worked to castrate the virus' DNA
and thus slow down its insidious takeover of healthy cells.
They also warned him that there are often side-effects to this
drug, including bone-marrow depression that leads to anaemia.

Reluctantly he agreed. He is an aware and very health-
conscious person, and intuited that if he were to take them at
all, he ought to be positive about it. So he dropped all resistance from the past in his mind to ''drugs'' and chose to see
them as his ''little helpers'' instead. Before taking them he
reminds himself that the pills are his friends, helping to keep
him alive, and he then feels gratitude to them. Each set he
takes he visualises as shift-workers going on duty—the last
four of the day he calls the ''night shift''—and he sends them
off to ''work'' with a blessing. He has programmed himself
not to have side-effects—and hasn't. Nearly a year after the
initial diagnosis of AIDS he is symptom-free, working, and,
he says, feeling as healthy as he ever has.

Martin Brofman told me once that one of the ways he helped to heal himself of cancer was to imagine, whenever he went to the toilet, that he was expelling cancerous cells from his body.

Penny Brohn also has some good ideas, "If you are gardening, focus your mind for a moment or two on the idea of the weed you are pulling up being a cancer cell. As you clear and aerate the soil, imagine your body doing the same thing . . . You could equally imagine your body being cleansed of cancer each time you hold a dirty plate under a running tap, or clean the bath, or put a load of washing in the machine." (*The Bristol Programme* see page 190). Healing yourself is a fulltime job.

Detoxifying Affirmations

With every outbreath I rid my body of toxins.
Every breath I take cleanses my body totally.

White Light Visualisation

As always before any visualisation, relax as deeply as you can: by lying down, taking a few deep breaths, clearing your mind in the ways shown in the Alpha Plan, and becoming more aware of your body.

Imagine you are surrounded by White Light. As you focus on it more and more, the Light becomes brighter and brighter. Know that this Light is purifying and healing. Allow it to enter your body through the top of your head. Feel it permeating throughout your body, as it does so clearing out all the dark corners, washing away any junk, any dirt, that has been stored there. Feel the Light flowing out through your feet, taking any old, stale and unhealthy energy with it. Continue until you feel totally "cleaned out," refreshed and revitalised.

Waterfall Visualisation

Whenever you take a shower, imagine that you are standing under a waterfall in the heart of a forest. It is a magic wa-

terfall, for the water has healing powers. As you stand under the shower, imagine that the water cascading down your body is cleansing you inside as well, washing away all impurities, all bacteria and viruses, leaving you fresh and clean within as well as without.

Remember with affirmations and visualisations that the more you believe what you affirm and the more you feel what you visualise, the more powerful the healing effect on your body.

Finally, a word about freshness. It is not accidental that we associate germs with dirt. We know they need it to flourish. But as well as merely keeping your body clean (for example by taking a daily shower, or at least a full body wash), also it is good to put on a fresh set of clothes each day.

Try in every way you can to freshen your vibrations and those around you. Make sure you air the sick-room regularly, that any soiled bed linen is immediately changed, that your bedside table is not allowed to stay too long a mess of banana skins and grape twigs, presided over by dead flowers. One of the reasons we traditionally bring fresh flowers to the sick is to sweeten the vibrations of the sickroom with their colours and their fragrance. Freshness is life.

And what also sweetens vibrations—perhaps above all else—is love. So welcome any loving energy into your sick room in whatever form it wants to come. Have handy some photographs of loved ones for you to look at, or, if you are religiously inclined, some images that evoke feelings in you of trust and love. These can be especially comforting, lit by the soft glow of a nightlight, in those wee small hours when you may not be able to sleep and the demons of depression and fear are on the loose.

eight

NOURISHING YOUR IMMUNE SYSTEM

As well as getting enough rest and detoxifying our bodies, nourishing ourselves properly when we are ill is supremely important. For many (especially people into macrobiotics) the "Way of Food" is *the* royal road to better health.

In this section we shall consider which nutrients have been found to strengthen our immune systems and how to ensure that we get enough of them. We shall start with vitamin C because the most spectacular healing claims have been made for this vitamin.

Vitamin C

Foods rich in this vitamin include: green and red peppers; green, leafy vegetables (e.g., broccoli, brussels sprouts, spinach); potatoes; cauliflower; cabbage; parsley; strawberries; and fresh citrus fruits (e.g., oranges, grapefruit).

It is something of a mystery why vitamin C has such healing and protective properties, for deficiency of it does not seem actually to affect the immune system itself. And yet it has been claimed to alleviate almost everything from the common cold and flu to cancer and AIDS. Its beneficent function seems to consist in its enhancement of phagocyte motility (white blood cell activity) and ability to deal with bacteria and fungi, probable promotion of the release of interferon (which attacks viruses), and its role as an anti-oxidant and free radical scavenger. It also helps to prevent the formation of carcinogens in the body.

Dr. Linus Pauling and Scottish cancer surgeon Ewan Cameron both recommend 10 grams a day of vitamin C as beneficial in some cases of cancer. The Californian orthopaedic surgeon Robert Cathcart is in favour of even higher doses—even up to 180 gms of intravenous vitamin C per 24 hours, supplemented with oral doses, for seriously ill AIDS patients. The more ill you are, he says, the more your body needs vitamin C. The maximum it will tolerate will be reached when diarrhoea sets in. It should then be reduced by around 20%, which will then be the optimum dose. Apparently even with these megadoses no cases of kidney stones have ever been reported.

It should once again be repeated that nowhere in this book are we suggesting self-treatment, so much as reporting the results of recent research into what works for healing and what doesn't. Even less is it intended to suggest that one should try to "go it alone" or abandon any prescribed treatment for vitamin C therapy. If you intend to take more than 1 or 2 grams of vitamin C daily as a supplement you should discuss this with your doctor first.

Beta-Carotene

This is the form of vitamin A most easily assimilated by the body. Vitamin A is found in green, leafy vegetables and in red and yellow fruits: carrots; spinach; watercress; apricots; broccoli; peaches; tomatoes; watermelon; cherries and asparagus are a particularly rich source. It is also found in fish (especially cod and halibut liver oil); liver; milk and dairy products. Munching one carrot a day is prophylactic, for it contains about 10,000 IU (International Units) of beta-carotene (nearly 7 times the RDA (Recommended Daily Allowance).

Vitamin A seems to be one of the most effective protective nutrients against cancer. It has also been found able to combat the suppression of the immune function that often follows surgery, so if you are recovering from an operation make sure you get enough of the vitamin. Patients in the Cohen study in 1979 given high daily doses showed heightened T cell activity a week after surgery as compared with a control group (who received no vitamin A) whose immune systems showed the usual post-surgery suppression.

Be warned, however, that it is easy to overdose on vitamin A. In fact this is the most common form of vitamin toxicity there is, due to the fact that this vitamin is oil-soluble and can accumulate in the body's fat cells. The patients in the Cohen study were given very large doses of 300,000 to 450,000 IU without registering any toxicity. But once again, as in the case of vitamin C megadosing, these should not be self-administered without consulting your doctor. Weiner suggests 20,000 to 100,000 IU per day as the supplement range. The Bristol Cancer Help Centre recommend taking carotene in the form of fresh carrot juice, about one to one and a half pints daily. Oil should be added (about a teaspoonful) to help assimilation by the body.

Vitamin B6 (pyrodoxine)

This appears to be the most important of all the B vitamins for strengthening the immune system, and deficiency can cause serious immune problems. B6 also helps to maintain good circulation and prevent heart disease. The following are sources of B6: bananas; avocados; tomatoes; onions; apples; asparagus; meat; whole grains; green vegetables (especially lettuce and spinach); peas; prunes; wheat germ; molasses and brewer's yeast.

Folic Acid

Deficiency of this B vitamin has been shown to depress immune functioning. It also assists red blood formation, so sufferers from anaemia should make sure they are getting enough. Signs of deficiency include anaemia, weakness, loss of appetite, fatigue and depression. Sources of this vitamin include; milk and dairy products; green, leafy vegetables (especially spinach, endive, brussels sprouts and broccoli); lentils; turnips; nuts; whole grains; soya beans; salmon; tuna; brewer's yeast; and potatoes (a 6 oz. portion provides half the RDA).

Pantothenic Acid

This vitamin promotes the formation of antibodies and is therefore very good for your immune system. As nutritionist Adele Davis reported long ago, pantothenic acid also plays an important role in reducing stress since it contains what she called rather mysteriously "stress factors." It is present in liver (which Ms. Davis recommends as part of a "stress diet" whenever we are really "going through it") and kidneys; salmon; wheat germ; whole grains; mushrooms; milk; egg yolks; leafy green vegetables; sprouting grains and seeds; sesame and sunflower seeds—and the ubiquitous brewer's yeast. It is in fact found in so many foods that deficiencies are rare.

Riboflavin (B2)

Like pantothenic acid, riboflavin also promotes antibody production and therefore is an immunity enhancer. Again, like folic acid, it assists in the formation of red blood cells. Note that this vitamin is destroyed by direct sunlight.

Riboflavin is found in: spinach; broccoli; brussels sprouts; asparagus; cauliflower; peas; green peppers; meat; soya beans; milk; cheese; wheat germ; whole grains; nuts—and brewer's yeast!

Vitamin B12 (Cobalamin)

Recent studies have suggested that this vitamin stimulates immune functioning and that a deficiency reduces T and B cell proliferation, blocking of immunoglobulins, and a reduction in the ability of the white cells to kill bacteria. Deficiency of B12 (and indeed of vitamin B generally) manifests often as irritability and "nerves." It is particularly important for vegetarians (and even more so, vegans) to ensure they get an adequate supply of B12, for, rather than in vegetables, this vitamin is found in fish and meat, eggs, milk and dairy products (e.g., cottage cheese).

Thiamin (B1)

Thiamin is less important for the immune system than the other B vitamins mentioned above, but deficiency has been correlated with the total number of T and B cells in the blood and immunoglobulin response. It is found in potatoes, spinach, cauliflower, asparagus, brussels sprouts, broccoli, peas, brown rice, nuts, wheat germ, meat and poultry—and, believe it or not, brewer's yeast.

Note: It is important to take the whole B complex rather than just a few of the B vitamins. *The Bristol Programme* (see page 190) recommends brewer's yeast as the best way of getting your B vitamins in supplement form. They suggest two tablets taken three times daily. Alternatively they recommend taking capsules of vitamin B complex (12,500 IU) twice a day. However, anyone suffering from candida should avoid taking any form of yeast and take multi-B vitamin capsules instead.

Vitamin E

This is similar to vitamin C in several ways. It is an effective antioxydant, stimulates the immune system, protects against infection, and is a scavenger of free radicals. It also protects cell membranes against lipid peroxidation. (Lipid peroxidation is a process undergone by polyunsaturated fats in the body, similar to the development of rancidity in oils. Liquid peroxidation releases dangerous free radicals—molecular fragments capable of damaging cells, causing genetic damage, and perhaps even causing cancer.) It helps to protect against cancer, blood clots, too high cholesterol levels, the effects of air pollution on the lungs, and the effects of stress generally. It is also credited with rejuvenating effects, restoring sexual energy and (applied externally as a cream) with clearing up skin ailments. No wonder it has been called the "wonder vitamin"!

Vitamin E is present in the following foods: dark green vegetables (e.g., spinach, broccoli, parsley); eggs; liver; kidneys; wheat germ; vegetable oils; asparagus; almonds; walnuts; seeds and whole grain cereals (one 4 oz serving of muesli provides a quarter of the RDA). Taken as a daily supplement, 100 IU would seem to be what most dieticians recommend.

Selenium

Taking selenium in conjunction with vitamin E seems to increase the effectiveness of both, for they work synergistically. It is only fairly recently that we have discovered how very important selenium is for the proper working of the immune system. Research carried out in 1984 revealed, in fact, that selenium is the most potent known anti-carcinogen there is. The preceding year it had been found that the incidence of tumours in animals was greatly reduced when they were given extra selenium, while Soviet researchers already knew that it increased antibody response in animals to a whole range of antigens. An article in the *British Medical Journal* for February 1985 reported that selenium deficiency might lead to a greater chance of developing cancer.

Selenium appears to increase the ability of our "fighting cells" to kill bacteria and attack tumours. Also, like the vitamin E with which it likes to work, it is a powerful antioxidant and prevents damage from free radicals and protects cell membranes from lipid peroxidation.

Yet of all the supplements discussed here, the most caution has to be exercised with selenium, for it is highly toxic when taken to excess. Foods containing selenium include: fish; whole grains; breads and cereals; wheat germ; milk; butter; garlic; and fruit and nuts.

Zinc

Like selenium, zinc is extremely important for good immune system functioning. It promotes the formation of T cells, and deficiency can reduce their number as well as causing atrophy of the all-important thymus. Zinc deficiency also makes for poor healing of burns and other wounds. Our body's store of zinc is depleted by eating too much fibre, drinking too much alcohol, and (for men) over-indulgence in sex to orgasm. (And, while we're on the subject of sex, the general consensus seems to be that physical intimacy with a loved one is beneficial for the seriously ill, e.g., AIDS and cancer patients. Actual sex, assuming they have the energy, should not, however, be indulged in to the point where physical exhaustion results. For men, ejaculation should be avoided, and if it occurs, the body's supply of zinc, which is lost with orgasm should be replenished with supplements.)

Sources of zinc include: seafood; liver; mushrooms; soya beans; spinach and sunflower seeds. Taken as a supplement the usual recommendation is 15mg daily. Weiner cautions against taking extra zinc if you have a bacterial or a candida infection because, though zinc increases T cell immunity, it has been shown to depress the function of the phagocytes. He suggests that, though zinc is known to promote wound healing, it might not be advisable to take it after surgery or burns as it might actually encourage bacterial infection. He also cautions against taking iron or vitamin D, which may actually *feed* the bacteria.

Summary

1. In our lists above the same foods keep turning up over and over again as containing the nutrients our immune systems need, especially if they are already depressed. These are the foods we should make our staple diet. They include:
     fresh vegetables, especially leafy green ones (remember, raw, steamed, or lightly cooked) like broccoli, spinach, brussels sprouts, carrots, potatoes, garlic and onion, and (if you can afford it) asparagus
     fruits, nuts and seeds
     fish (a few times a week)
     whole grains
     wheat germ
     eggs (sparingly)
     milk and soft cheeses

liver or kidneys (occasionally)

vegetable oil (preferably olive oil or grapeseed oil)

2. Care should be exercised when taking supplements. Some vitamins work synergistically (which means behaving as a catalyst for each other) and it is important to maintain a correct balance. It is easy to get confused about dosages and it is possible to overdose to the point of toxicity (especially in the case of vitamin A and selenium). The RDA is not much help, since it is outdated. These "Recommended Daily Allowances" were set up during the Second World War as guidelines for the *minimum* nutritional requirements for mass-feeding programmes. On the other hand we have reports of the spectacular results being achieved with megadoses of, for example, vitamin C. And, certainly in the case of patients with severely damaged immune systems (e.g., cancer, AIDS) it is *essential* that immunity be boosted with, for example, vitamin C, the B vitamins, zinc and selenium.

It would obviously therefore be useful to know exactly what one is deficient in and by how much before setting up a programme of supplements. This is possible by going to the trouble of getting a personal blood analysis done. Alternatively, consult a practitioner of kinesiology who will work out what supplements you need via a technique that registers muscle strength in response to various nutrients placed on the body (usually the navel). It sounds weird but apparently is effective in showing what the body needs (and also what it is allergic to), and is an interesting example of how we can enlist the body's own innate intelligence and wisdom to tell us what it needs.

Kinesiology is a therapy to do with touch, not as in manipulative or postural processes, but as a way of transmitting or arousing healing energy in the body. One such system (called Applied Kinesiology) works via specific muscle-testing techniques to discover weaknesses and to correct them. Each group of muscles is related to one of the acupuncture meridians. The system was developed by Dr. George Goodhart, a Detroit chiropractor and introduced into Britain by Brian Butler. Butler runs courses for lay people (called ''Touch for Health''—see Appendix) in which he teaches them how to detect and correct muscle imbalances for themselves. Kinesiology is most widely used today to discover nutritional requirements and to test for food allergies.

Contact addresses, if you want to enlist professional help in sorting out your specific nutritional requirements, are listed in the Resources appendix (on page 193). Finally, in Part 3, we shall be giving nutritional guidelines to those wrestling with keeping the HIV virus at bay (at whatever stage) and examining what AIDS sufferers are doing to heal themselves and to complement whatever help they are managing to get from a beleaguered medical establishment.

nine

BOOSTING YOUR
VITAL ENERGY

Whatever our illness, whatever symptoms we may be suffering from, one of them is almost certainly to be feeling that we don't have any energy. We tend to feel "washed out," tired, easily fatigued. In this section we examine what else can be done, as well as relaxing and nourishing ourselves properly, to help bring some life and energy back into our bodies. And when we raise our store of "chi" or "prana" we raise our spirits too. For how we experience life is always a reflection of our energy-levels: when we say we are feeling "low" (or "high") we are really talking about how much vitality we have, how much of the life-force is flowing through us.

In this connection we might first mention the energy-boosting dietary supplements that you might like to add to the immune-enhancers just recommended in the preceding chapter.

SPECIAL SUPPLEMENTS

Ginseng

This interesting root has enjoyed recognition as a medical plant in the Far East for over 4,000 years. There they call it "the root of life." Chinese doctors still prescribe it today for loss of vigour (including sexual potency), anaemia, nervous disorders and insomnia. Ginseng is such a powerful energy booster that it should not be taken late in the day or it could stop you from sleeping. The Russians apparently give it to astronauts on space missions to heighten their alertness, energy and endurance.

Ginseng grows only in a few dry and mountainous areas of the world, for example Siberia and Korea. It takes six to seven years before the roots can be harvested, which is why it is a little on the expensive side. But it is so rich in nutrients, minerals and trace elements that it is worth investing in. Ginseng appears on the market in the form of the root itself, as tea, or in capsules of varying potency.

Note: Ginseng should only be taken over short periods by women as it stimulates the male hormones. The Chinese list it as a "yang," or masculine food. It is, therefore, a "male" remedy, and is less appropriate for women except in cases of extremely low energy levels, and then not for prolonged use. Ginseng should certainly not be used by women with menstrual or menopausal difficulties. It should also be treated with caution in the case of prostatic disease in men.

Calcium Supplements

If you are feeling strained and irritable, you could well be short of calcium. Try boosting your calcium intake with calcium lactate over a short period. It is obtainable from high street chemists, usually in 300mg strength. Calcium pantothenate is also effective when feeling stressed.

Royal Jelly

Some people I know swear by this, admittedly expensive, food manufactured by bees for their queen. Like ginseng, it is full of vitamins, trace elements, and amino acids and is a great energy-booster. Treat yourself to some!

EXERCISE

One of the main ways we can raise our energy when we are well is by taking exercise. Not, of course, so easy though when you are ill, especially if you are ill in bed. And yet another proof of the power of visualisation has been the discovery that merely *imagining* that you are exercising produces some of the benefits of real exercise in the body. So lie back and enjoy a leisurely swim in your local pool, or a jog in the park, and feel that it's doing you good. That said, if it is at all possible, try to get up and stay up as long as you can without exhausting yourself. Take a stroll up and down the hospital corridor to exercise those legs, which are the first muscles to show signs of wasting if you don't give them something to do. There comes a point at which we start to lose energy rather than gain it by staying in bed for too long. Exercise those muscles in any way you can, if only by flexing and relaxing them periodically under the sheets. Here are some bed exercises:

1. Some hospitals have a triangle over the bed which you can use to lift the upper part of your body up and down, and thus exercise your arms, shoulders and back. Alternatively, this can be done holding on to the head of the bed.

2. Belly muscles can be toned by alternatively tensing and relaxing them. This should be done only on an empty stomach and after breathing out.

3. Bring the knees up to the belly in an umbilical position. Hold, straighten legs again, and repeat.

4. Move feet up and down from the ankle repeatedly during the day. Restores circulation and prevents blood clots and gangrene. For the same reason, *never* cross your feet at the ankles. (Also refer to Massage, below).

MASSAGE

Try and get someone in to massage you, every day if possible. There are several forms of massage to choose from; some relax, some balance energy, and some invigorate. Depending on how fragile you are feeling (and also whether you have specific tensions in any part of your body that you would like eased away) you may opt for any of them on any particular day.

Particularly energy-boosting is the type of massage called *shiatsu* which works on acupressure points to stimulate nerves and circulation and tone muscles. Be warned, however, that shiatsu can be quite painful if you are in bad shape, in which case settle for the gentler form aimed at making you feel more relaxed and in your body. And remember that your masseur (or masseuse) need not necessarily be professionally trained. Anyone who loves you and wants you to get well will probably do a marvellous job if they trust their intuition and let their hands guide them. Touch is healing—and a loving touch most of all.

In the absence of somebody else to massage you, massage yourself to get the energy moving in and to tone muscles. Massaging oneself is very natural; we do it all the time (albeit maybe unconsciously) to help ourselves feel better. For example, we scratch our heads when perplexed, instinctively rub bumps and bruises, press on insect bites . . .

Obviously you won't be able to give yourself the full body massage somebody else can give you. But here's what you *can* do:

Hand Massage

Rub your hands vigorously together. Apart from anything else, you will be energising them for massaging other parts of your body. Pull each finger from the base to the tip, using the thumb and index finger of the opposite hand, and finishing each stroke with a snap. Grasp one hand with the other in any way that feels good and squeeze it firmly with a stroking motion. Alternate with each hand. Use the thumb to smooth the palm of the other hand.

Belly Palming

Rub the belly firmly with the palm of your hand in a *clockwise* motion (to follow the direction of digestion in the colon). This, incidentally, is a good thing to do if you are constipated. Also, an energy-boosting exercise from Chinese yoga is to rub vigorously, up and down, the area between the navel and the pubis. This area, called in Japanese the "hara," is considered in the East to be the centre of our vital energy, which you will thus be stimulating.

Arm Meridian Massage

Massaging along the lines of the acupuncture meridians boosts the flow of energy along them and invigorates. But make sure you follow the flow as follows. With the *right* hand, rub the whole length of the *left* arm, from the back of the left hand up the outside of the arm to the left shoulder, then (in one continuous stroke) down the inside of the left arm to the palm of the left hand. Use brisk, firm strokes, applying a constant pressure and finishing up with a flick—as if you were brushing off drops of water from your fingers. Do this half a dozen times or so. Repeat the sequence on the right arm using the left hand.

Leg Meridian Massage

The energy flow along the meridians in the legs is in the opposite direction to that in the arms. So stroke briskly *down* the outside of the legs from hip to ankles and *up* the inside of the legs as far as the upper inside thighs, in one flowing movement. Both legs can be massaged simultaneously, using the left hand for the left leg and right hand for the right leg.

Eye Palming

Particularly good if you are feeling drained by too much going on around you and need to withdraw from sensory stimulation for a while. Place the palms lightly over the eyes, fingers crossed on the forehead. *Do not press on the eyeball itself.* Close your eyes, relax, and let your eyeballs sink deep into their sockets. Keep your palms over your eyes until you feel ready to come out and face the world again. This is also one of the main Bates exercises for improving eyesight. Dr. William H. Bates (1881–1931) published *Better Eyesight Without Glasses* in 1919, which became a bestseller in the USA. He was an eye specialist and an instructor at the New York Postgraduate Medical School, and he challenged the assumption that eyesight must necessarily deteriorate with age, and suggested that in fact wearing glasses made your eyes weaker. The Bates Method consists of a series of exercises to strengthen the eye muscles so that the lens is brought back into "true" naturally, rather than adjusting itself to seeing through an artificial lens. The exercises include "palming" the eyes (i.e., relaxing the eyes by covering them gently with the palms); splashing the closed eyes for 20 minutes morning and night (warm water in the morning, cold water at night); near and far focussing, alternatively, on two pencils held in either hand—one held about 15cm from your nose—the other held at arm's length in a direct line behind it, and so on.

Face Massage

One of the most soothing things you can do for yourself (applying hot face flannels, or soaking your wrists in hot water are others). Here's how. Rub your hands vigorously together to warm them, then bring that energy to your face by placing your hands over it, fingers over the eyes. Smooth the forehead firmly, using the two middle fingers of both hands simultaneously. Start the strokes from the middle of the forehead and end at the temples. After a while, switch your attention to your jaw, where we usually tend to hold a lot of tension. Applying very firm pressure, trace the line of the upper jaw from each side of the nostrils to down to the sides of the mouth. Place the second and third fingers on each side of the jaw and clench the latter. Shift the position of the fingers if necessary so that they are right over the tensed jaw muscle. Then relax the jaw and rub as hard as is comfortable, using small circular strokes.

Scalp Massage

Apply friction to the scalp with the fingertips, rubbing and tapping—be firm but gentle.

Foot Massage

Finish up with this as it takes more time. Massaging your feet is ideal when fatigued and is very relaxing and soothing. Sit in any comfortable position which will allow you to massage the sole of each foot in turn. Make a fist and press the knuckles hard into the ball of each foot, using a "screwing" motion. Do the same with the instep. Make a ring with thumb and index finger, insert each toe in turn through it and pull firmly with a wriggling stroke. Pinch the tip of each toe. Rub the index finger between each toe. Using the second fingers, smooth the hollows on each side of the Achilles tendon in a downward direction. Pinch the heel a few times sharply. Finish with grasping one foot with both hands from the sides, thumbs overlapping toes. Press with the fingers into the sole, meanwhile smoothing the top of the foot forward with the fleshy part of each palm. Repeat with the other foot.

ZONE THERAPY (REFLEXOLOGY)

Massaging the hands and feet is not only soothing for the nerves and invigorating, but also healing. When we do so we are also stimulating the internal organs and increasing circulation to and energising all the areas of the body, not just the hands and feet. It is not clear why this should be so. Reflexologists believe that each part of the hands and feet corresponds with various organs of the body, and by stimulating the nerve endings in the former one can send healing energy to the latter. The approximate position of these nerve endings and the parts to which they correspond and which will be energised by their manipulation have been charted and are given in the "maps" on pages 94–95.

The exact "reflex area" for each organ may vary slightly

Reflexology Map of the Hands

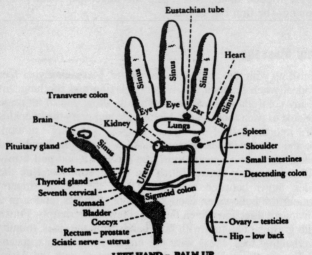

LEFT HAND – PALM UP

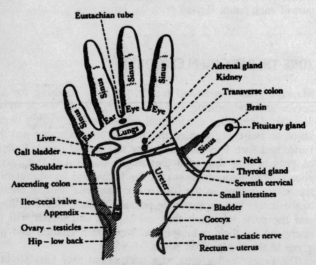

RIGHT HAND – PALM UP

Reflexology Map of the Feet

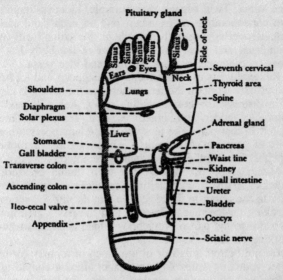

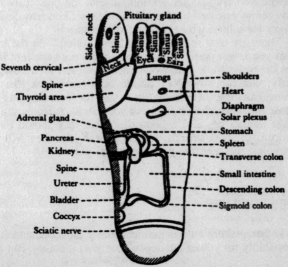

from person to person. Note that those on the left hand and
left foot correspond to organs on the left side of the body, and
vice versa. Twin organs (for example, kidneys, lungs) have
two corresponding reflex areas, one on each hand and foot.
Organs overlapping both sides (e.g., the colon) will overlap
each hand and foot. The upper part of the body has reflex
areas on the upper parts of the foot and vice versa.

Reflexologists use these maps for diagnosis and for healing,
and usually work on the feet rather than the hands. If an organ
is in distress, the corresponding reflex area will tend to be
painful or tender, and sometimes small gravelly nodules can
be felt in that part. The less you can tolerate pressure on the
soles of your feet (for example, when walking barefoot across
a pebbly beach), the worse shape your internal organs are in.

Manipulating the tender area with thumb pressure (and
knuckles to disperse crystalline deposits) sends nourishing energy to the organ in distress. You can do this for yourself by
checking on the maps where to find the reflex area that corresponds to the part of your body which is under stress—and
working on it.

Do not be too rough or in too much of a hurry for results.
After your first reflexology massage, allow a couple of days
before you try another session, so that the body can absorb
any toxins released into the bloodstream. (You may feel a bit
dizzy for a little while but this soon passes.)

There are also small wooden "foot rollers" on the market
that you might prefer to use. You simply put each foot in turn
on the roller—and roll away, backwards and forwards. Similarly, you can buy spiky plastic balls (they look like small
mines) and use them in the same way (or for massaging those
tense and unreachable places in your back). Acupressure massage sandals are also a good idea—but they should only be
worn over short periods, not permanently, or they will over-
stimulate the reflexology and pressure points.

ACUPUNCTURE

Whether making an appointment to see an acupuncturist is a
possibility for you or not depends on your mobility. But if you

have got over the worst of your illness, and are convalescing, it would be very worthwhile considering investing in a series of sessions with a qualified acupuncturist. Of all the therapies, acupuncture is the one that works most directly on unblocking, redirecting and balancing our energy and this is precisely what is needed in order to get well again—whatever you may be suffering from. Surgery, in particular, is a drastic intervention in the body's subtle energy layers, often cutting across the path of energy meridians. So acupuncture is definitely to be recommended if you have had a major operation, in order to speed total recovery from the trauma to which the body has been subjected.

Acupuncture receives most publicity perhaps for its known capacity to relieve pain. In China (where it has been used for 5,000 years and now complements orthodox medicine), it is sometimes used as an alternative to anaesthetic in surgical operations. In 1979 in China, over 3 million such operations were performed, with no deaths reported. In Munich, too, acupuncture has been used in more than 2,000 operations at the German Heart Centre as a way of reducing the amount of drugs administered to anaesthetised patients.

In Britain, many National Health Service pain clinics have been using acupuncture on patients with migraines, backaches and so forth when they have not responded to conventional drugs or surgery.

Recent research has suggested that acupuncture relieves pain because it causes endorphins to be released into the spinal fluid. (First discovered in 1975, endorphins are chemicals produced by the pituitary gland which have a similar effect to morphine in relieving pain and changing moods. They are released in moments of stress, which is why sportsmen or soldiers, for example, are able to carry on as if nothing has happened, when in fact they may have been quite seriously injured). If, therefore, one reason why you are feeling drained is because you are in constant pain you may well explore what an acupuncturist can do for you.

ACUPRESSURE

In the meantime, before trying acupuncture, you could try some acupressure on yourself. This, like acupuncture, works on the pressure points along the energy meridian, but without needles. These points have all been given numbers for ease of identification. There are certain points which you can press to get temporary relief from tension states, headache, fatigue, depression—even toothache until you can get to a dentist (I always use "large intestine 1" when I am in the dentist's chair while I am being injected, drilled or scaled. It really does work).

The acupressure technique is very simple. Use the tip of the thumb to apply firm pressure (about as much as you would use to make an indentation in a ball of clay). Press on the point for ten seconds, then press again for another ten seconds. Don't overdo it—and stop when you start to feel better. The corresponding point on the other side of the body should also be stimulated in the same way afterwards. Do NOT use acupressure, however, if you fall into the following categories:

• if you have heart trouble

• if you are on drugs or medication

• if you are in the last stages of pregnancy

• after a hot bath

• after a meal

• if the pressure point is on an open wound, scar, wart or mole.

These conditions would make the use of acupressure inadvisable because acupressure *stimulates* energy. This should not run counter to the body's own rhythms (e.g., the natural tendency to want to rest after a hot bath, or the depletion of energy due to being on drugs). Also, pressing hard on vulnerable (wounded or blemished) skin tissue is *not* a good idea.

Finding the exact point needs a certain amount of preliminary probing, for its exact location varies slightly with individuals—and it must be pressed in exactly the right place for anything to happen. So don't just press "somewhere in that

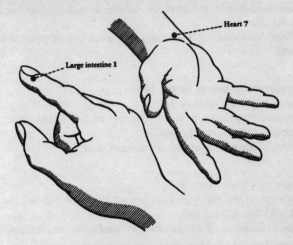

ACUPRESSURE POINTS

area,'' find the exact point by probing until you come across a slight indentation and feel a twinge. That's it. Here are some points to start off with. You will find other points in books listed under Further Reading (see page 190).

Acupressure Points in the Hands
Name of point: Heart **7**.
Location: The hollow in the crease on the side of the wrist (palm facing up) in line with the little finger.
Effect: Sedative. Use to combat insomnia, anxiety, irritability, depression.

Name of point: Large intestine **1**.
Location: Inside bottom corner of the nail of the finger of the right hand.
Effect: Tonic: against exhaustion, irritability. (This is also the point mentioned earlier that numbs toothache temporarily. Press the point on the same hand as the side the toothache is on.)

Acupressure Points in the Legs
Name of point: Stomach **36**.

Location: Below the kneecap, on the outside of the leg next to the shin bone.
Effect: Invigorating; for stimulating a feeling of general well-being.

Acupressure points in the Feet
Name of point: Kidney **3**.
Location: Midway between the top of the ankle bone and Achilles tendon, on the *inside*.
Effect: Sedative: against nervousness, fear.

Name of point: Liver **3**.
Location: One and a half inches up from the join of the big toe and the second toe.
Effect: Sedative: good for tension headaches and irritability.

PRANYAMA

These breathing exercises are taken from hatha yoga. As well as being energy boosters, they are also great mood-changers whenever you are feeling down and depressed.

Breathing Exercise 1

Stand in a relaxed posture, feet shoulder-width apart. Breathe in as deeply as you can, raising your arms in front of you as you do. Time it so that your arms are directly above your head as you complete the inhalation. Hold the breath for a count of five. Expel the air through your mouth with a deep sigh, allowing the arms to fall to either side and the shoulders to sag. Repeat as often as feels right but do not force it, especially if your chest is weak in some way. If it sounds too strenuous for you, you can do this exercise with the arms kept behind the back, and the hands joined together.

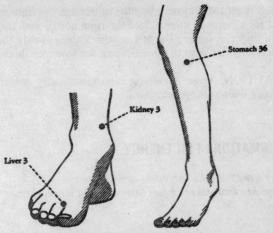

ACUPRESSURE POINTS

Breathing Exercise 2

Sitting or kneeling comfortably, inhale deeply through the nostrils. Imagine you are inhaling air first into the lower belly and feel the air filling you up inside like a balloon until it reaches the top of your chest. Hold for a few moments ONLY, then exhale slowly, imagining the "balloon" being deflated as air is expelled gently from the top of the chest down to the lower belly. As you inhale, imagine that you are taking in positive energy. Symbolise this energy to yourself in any way that is meaningful for you: as health, love, freshness, grace, or life, for example. As you exhale, imagine that you are expelling your fatigue, worries, sickness or anything else that is on your mind and burdening you.

Breathing Exercise 3

Close the right nostril with the right index finger. Breathe in deeply through the left nostril. Hold for a count of three. Close the left nostril with the left index finger, removing the right finger from the right nostril and exhale. Count to three. With the left nostril still closed, breathe in through the right nostril. Hold for a count of three. Close the right nostril with the right index finger, releasing the left nostril. Exhale slowly through the left nostril. Count to three. Repeat the sequence three times only.

CAUTION: Yogic breathing is extraordinarily powerful— so don't overdo these exercises.

AFFIRMATIONS FOR ENERGY

Every breath I take increases my aliveness.
Every day that passes I feel stronger and more alive.

VISUALISATIONS FOR ENERGY

Exercise

See yourself enjoying your favourite form of exercise when you were well. The more strenuous it is, the more energy you will get from this visualisation. If your choice is tennis, for example, see yourself serving at full strength, belting the ball from the baseline . . . forehand, backhand . . . cross-court, down the line . . . Remember the satisfaction you felt when you were hitting it hard and in the centre of the racket, watching it speed low over the net and deep into the corners . . . See your opponent wilting under the pressure and returning a ball short . . . You race up to the net and punch a killing volley that leaves him (or her) totally wrong-footed . . . Or maybe you are swimming in your local pool, length after length . . . Remember the euphoria of the rhythmic strokes, steady breathing . . . Treat yourself to a sauna afterwards and feel your skin tingling in the dry heat, and how relaxed and alive you feel . . . Any form of exercise will do. The important thing, as ever, is to actually get the feel in your body that this is all really happening.

Chakras Visualisation

Let your attention rest in your First Chakra (see page 33), i.e., in the general area of the buttocks). Relax, and allow yourself to feel any sensations that want to be experienced. Breathe into this area. Start to imagine the colour red, in any way that it wants to come . . . red curtains, a red scarf—or just a red haze. Continue to feel your first chakra area as you create red in your mind's eye. Feel the lower part of your body vibrating with this colour . . . After a few minutes, when it feels right, let your attention move up to the area just above the genitals—the Second Chakra. Allow yourself a few moments to tune into whatever sensations you are experiencing in this area—and relax and breathe into them . . . Now create the colour orange in your imagination. See this colour surrounding you—or visualise a bowl of oranges, an orange beach ball, anything orange . . . Enjoy the colour orange for as long as you want, then move on up the chakras in turn. Give yourself plenty of time. There is no hurry. With each chakra, follow the same technique; tune into that part of the body, feel what sensations are there in that area, breathe and relax into them, and imagine as clearly and as brightly as you can the colour associated with that particular chakra. Remember the chart of the chakras on page 34. Here are the other chakras and colours:

> *Solar plexus (yellow)*
> *Heart (green)*
> *Throat (blue)*
> *"Third eye" (indigo)*
> *Crown of the head (violet)*

When you have done the seventh chakra, finish by visualising yourself surrounded by white light (which contains all the other colours). Give more and more attention to this white light so that it becomes brighter and brighter, clearer and clearer . . . Allow it to enter your body, to fill you out, every nook and cranny . . . Feel it warming and nourishing you, cleansing you, washing away every impurity, germ, toxin, bringing freshness and light to any dark places that you intuit may be there . . . Enjoy this purifying and energising visualisation for as long as you want, for it is healing you at a very deep level.

ten

LETTING GO OF NEGATIVITY

Why is it so important, especially if we are ill, to let go of negativity? The short answer is that hanging on to it does us no good at all and very probably helped to make us ill in the first place. By contrast, making a deliberate choice to let go of negative mental patterns, as we have seen, definitely improves our health, sometimes quite dramatically. Quite apart from whether acid thoughts create acid blood, or whether fear exhausts the immune system, hanging on to negativity takes a lot of energy that would be more usefully employed in healing the beleaguered body rather than maintaining it permanently in a state of readiness for "fight or flight."

So do yourself a favour. Choose to forgive rather than to keep re-creating the old resentments, brooding over the hurts, re-running the old movies. To forgive does not mean to condone what may have been done to you in the past, it simply means to let go of it. And the quickest way to let go of something is if you see how holding on to it is hurting you in the present. We let go instinctively, automatically, of something we pick up that burns our hand, while cooking, for example. We spit out immediately food we have put into our mouths that tastes bad. We don't need to think about it, we just do it, in the interests of self-preservation. Think of a negative mental pattern in the same way; as something you took on board when you didn't know any better, when perhaps the only way of reacting to being hurt was to hate. But now you know what a little time bomb you have been carrying around inside you or, to change the image, how you have been toxifying your whole system. However, you can do something about it. Very simply get rid of it. Just drop it.

RELEASING NEGATIVE FEELING

This is not as hard as it sounds. It is simply a choice. The good news is that you don't have to become a saint overnight. Your subconscious will respond to even just an affirmation that you are *willing* to forgive, even if you don't really feel that you are there yet. The more you affirm forgiveness, the more the feeling of forgiveness will grow in you and become your new reality. As Caroline Myss puts it, "Fake it till you make it." Louise Hay assures us that it does not matter how long a negative "tape" has been with us, or even if we're not exactly clear as to what particular brand of negativity is recorded on it. Our body will respond to new programming of our subconscious, to the change in us from being contracted, "uptight," perhaps revengeful, to being more forgiving, accepting, loving. At the very least we will feel more relaxed about things.

Remember that our "past" is always our creation, and we can make it anything we want by our selective memory of certain facts and ignoring others. So you think you had a rotten childhood. But surely there must have been *some* good times sometimes? But if one is determined to be a victim one will always be able to ferret out the "facts" to support the status. And Life always supports us totally in what we choose to believe is true about ourselves—and provides the experiences to match.

Let us be clear that we are not saying that one should never get angry, or that one should deny one's fear. There may be perfectly valid reasons for feeling either of these primary emotions based on objective considerations. On the contrary, these feelings *in the moment* must always be acknowledged, whether or not we choose to act them out—and in a later section (see page 183) we shall be looking at how important it is that we give ourselves permission to express our feelings as much as we can. What we are talking about here are habitual ingrained patterns of negativity that we carry around with us all the time: resentment (which is anger energy going nowhere, frozen into the body); depression and guilt (anger turned against the self); continuous anxiety (fear that we refuse to confront head on); and grieving that goes on too long (refusal to say goodbye, mixed usually with anger at being abandoned). The most dangerous of them all is self-criticism. This is so crucial that we shall be devoting a special section later on (see page 128), to seeing how to get rid of this potentially lethal mental tape and programme ourselves for a healthy self-image.

Affirmations Which are Antidotes to Negative Mental Patterns

I have let go of any mental pattern which is creating negative effects in my life.

I am willing to forgive anyone who has ever hurt me, and wish them well.

I forgive X with all my heart and wish him (her, them) well.

I have let go of the past and now live totally in the present.

I trust that everything happened as it was meant to, and that all is well.

I forgive myself for holding on to negativity, and now let go of it.

VISUALISATIONS AGAINST NEGATIVITY

"Letting Go of Fear" Visualisation

See fear as a black cloud that is hovering over your head. There is a string that connects it with you. See yourself letting go of the string. Watch the black cloud as it floats away into the sky. Watch it getting smaller and smaller until it is just a speck—and eventually you cannot see it any more.

"Letting Go of Grief" Visualisation

See the person or scenes from the relationship over which you have been grieving too long. Allow yourself to really feel the pain of loss. Where in your body do you feel the hurt? Try to isolate the components of what you are feeling . . . is there anger there? Some guilt perhaps? How exactly were things left unfinished between you? What wasn't said that needed to be said? See yourself saying these things now to the person. Be absolutely honest and speak from the heart. Pause for a while and listen to the other's response. What is their message to you? Allow yourself to feel whatever you are feeling—and give yourself plenty of space for this . . . Stay with whatever comes up (however unexpected) until you feel "finished." Then, as gently and as lovingly as you can, say goodbye.

Metta Visualisation

Metta means "loving kindness" and is a Buddhist meditation. It is an example of "meditating on the opposite" to what you are feeling in order to stop fuelling negative thoughts and thereby re-creating negative feelings, and to create instead more positive energy by choosing to think loving thoughts.

Imagine that you are breathing out all tension, worry and negativity and breathing in patience, kindness and forgiveness. After a few moments of this, visualise your breath as light (either white or pink) that spreads throughout your body. Feel it warming and cleansing you . . . Now see this light spreading out from your body to envelop other people. This light is the energy carried by your good wishes for them, your "wishing them well." Extend it first to those you love who you know love you . . . Take your time, and include everybody you can think of who is close to you.

Now choose to include in your light those who, for whatever reason, you do not feel so kindly about, perhaps because you consider they have harmed you or behaved badly to you in the past. Remember, if you feel resistance to this, that you are not condoning what they did but acknowledging who they are, divine beings (however misguided) like yourself, fellow beings on this planet of ours. Don't suppress any resentment, that will probably still be there. Include it in the way you feel about that person—and choose to go beyond it and wish them well anyway. Remember that you are not doing it for them, you are doing it for **you** so that you can get well again. By choosing to love them, you are in fact showing your love for yourself. Finally, direct your light of compassion throughout the world, to all those others out there whom you do not know personally, but who may be suffering, like you, from ill-health or pain, or poverty, hunger, desperation, injustice and persecution . . . And finish up with loving yourself, and especially if you catch yourself judging yourself for not feeling as loving as you "should" be . . .

In the next few chapters we shall be looking in more depth at affirmations and visualisations since they are so important.

THE BACH FLOWER REMEDIES

To help dispel negativity, you could also take one of the Bach Flower Remedies. Make your selection, depending on which particular brand of negativity you are stuck in, from the following list. In the Appendix at the end of the book you can find out where to get them from. Fortunately, they are cheap. To quote from the official Dr. E. Bach Centre literature, "As the Bach Remedies are benign in their action and can result in no unpleasant reactions, they can be taken by anyone."

Stock Concentrate Remedies will keep indefinitely—a 10ml size concentrate bottle will prove sufficient to make approximately 60 treatment bottles. More than one Remedy can be taken at the same time—2 drops of each chosen Remedy should be diluted in a cup of water and sipped at intervals, or in a 30ml (1 fl. oz) bottle filled with spring water (this represents a treatment bottle) from which 4 drops are taken directly on the tongue at least 4 times a day. The "Rescue Remedy" is taken orally (4 drops in water) but can also be applied externally either in liquid or in cream form. Dr. Bach saved a fisherman's life in 1930 with this preparation.

The 39 Remedies

1. *Agrimony:* For those who suffer considerable inner torture which they try to dissemble behind a facade of cheerfulness.

2. *Aspen:* For apprehension—the feeling that something dreadful is going to happen without knowing why.

3. *Beech:* For those who are critical and intolerant of others, or arrogant.

4. *Centaury:* For weakness of will; those who let themselves be exploited or imposed upon—who become subservient and have difficulty saying "No." Human doormat.

5. *Cerato:* For those who doubt their own judgement and seek the advice of others. Often wrongly influenced and misguided.

6. *Cherry Plum:* For uncontrolled, irrational thoughts.

7. *Chestnut Bud:* Counteracts refusal to learn by experience, and continual repetition of the same mistakes.

8. *Chicory:* For the over-possessive person who demands respect or attention (selfishness), and likes others to conform to their standards. Those who make martyrs of themselves.

9. *Clematis:* For those who are indifferent, inattentive, dreamy, absent-minded. Mental escapists from reality.

10. *Crab Apple:* A cleanser. For those feeling unclean or ashamed of ailments. Self-disgust/hatred. For the house-proud.

11. *Elm:* For temporary feelings of inadequacy, those overwhelmed by responsibilities, but normally very capable.

12. *Gentian:* For the despondent who are easily discouraged and dejected.

13. *Gorse:* For despair and hopelessness, utter despondency and the feeling of "What's the use?".

14. *Heather:* For people who are obsessed with their own troubles and experiences, talkative "bores" and poor listeners.

15. *Holly:* For those who are jealous, envious, vengeful and suspicious, and for those who hate.

16. *Honeysuckle:* For those with nostalgic feelings who constantly dwell in the past, and for homesickness.

17. *Hornbeam:* For those with that "Monday morning feeling," who suffer from procrastination. However, once they have started, the task is usually fulfilled.

18. *Impatiens:* For the impatient and the irritable.

19. *Larch:* For those who are despondent through lack of self-confidence, and expectation of failure, so they fail to make the attempt. Feelings of inferiority, although they have the ability.

20. *Mimulus:* For the fear of known things. Shyness, timidity.

21. *Mustard:* For deep gloom or depression that descends for no known cause and lifts just as suddenly. Melancholy.

22. *Oak:* For those brave determined types who struggle on against adversity despite setbacks, the plodders.

23. *Olive:* For those who are drained of energy, and find everything an effort. For fatigue.

24. *Pine:* For feelings of guilt, those who blame themselves for the mistakes of others. Feelings of unworthiness.

25. *Red Chestnut:* For those who care too much and have excessive concern for others, especially those held dear.

26. *Rock Rose:* For those who are alarmed, scared, panicky, and full of trepidation.

27. *Rock Water:* For those who are hard on themselves—who often overwork, and are rigid minded, and self-denying.

28. *Scleranthus:* For those who feel uncertainty, indecision, or vacillation, and those with fluctuating moods.

29. *Star of Bethlehem:* For all the effects of serious news, or fright following an accident, etc.

30. *Sweet Chestnut:* For total dejection.

31. *Vervain:* For over-enthusiasm, over-effort, and straining. For those who overreach themselves and are fanatical and highly-strung, incensed and frustrated by injustices.

32. *Vine:* For the dominating, inflexible, ambitious, tyrannical, and autocratic. For those with arrogant pride, and those considered to be good leaders.

33. *Walnut:* A protection remedy from powerful influences— helps adjustment to any transition or change e.g., puberty, menopause, divorce, new surroundings.

34. *Water Violet:* Proud, reserved, sedate types, sometimes with a superior air. Those who have little emotional involvement but are reliable/dependable.

35. *White Chestnut:* For those with persistent unwanted thoughts, who are preoccupied with some worry or episode, or mental arguments.

36. *Wild Oat:* Helps to determine one's intended path in life.

37. *Wild Rose:* For those who feel resignation, or apathy. Drifters who accept their lot, making little effort for improvement, and lacking ambition.

38. *Willow:* For those who feel resentment and bitterness who take a "not fair" and "poor me" attitude.

39. *Rescue Remedy:* A combination of Cherry Plum, Clematis, Impatiens, Rock Rose and Star of Bethlehem. Rescue Remedy is an all-purpose emergency composite for shock, terror, panic, emotional upsets, "stage fright," examina-

tion, operations, dentistry, etc. Can also be externally applied to burns, bites, sprains and so on. Comforting, calming and reassuring to those distressed by startling experiences.

eleven

AFFIRMING THE POSITIVE

It cannot be too strongly emphasised that we must, in the words of the old Johnny Mercer song, "Accentuate the positive, eliminate the negative," if we are to get well again. However false it feels, however much it seems to go "against the grain," we must make the effort (and sometimes it feels like a gigantic effort) to lever ourselves out of the morass of depression, despair, self-pity, inner rage and self-destructiveness that sometimes threatens to engulf us, especially when we are feeling particularly weak and vulnerable. There is absolutely nothing to be got from giving in to these negative feelings— except more of them. The more we fuel them, the more they will grow. And the more toxic our bodies become, the more depressed our immunity, as we pump more and more adrenalin and corticoids into our system.

What we tell ourselves is supremely important. We are creating our future by what we think, say and feel NOW. The meanings we give to events, the conclusions we draw about "the way it is," the comparisons we make between ourselves and others, the image we are left with about ourselves, the past we create and the future we imagine—these become our reality, or rather, the filter in our minds through which we will interpret the outer reality.

"Facts" only have the meaning we give them, and there are as many "realities" as there are people. If we are programmed to see in a certain way, that is all we will see, or experience as "real." We will filter out anything that does not "fit" our programme, and attract the sorts of experiences to match the vibrations we are putting out, which will fulfil our own expectations of what is likely to happen. And Life will support us in anything we choose to believe is true about ourselves. It is tremendously respectful of our freedom to choose heaven or hell for ourselves.

Attention is energy. Whatever we give our attention to we get more of, and make more manifest and real for ourselves. The body is so constructed that it can see no difference between "real" reality and "imagined" reality. It reacts in the same way to either. If you think you have stepped on a venomous snake in the dark, the adrenalin will rush. You may laugh at your foolishness when you switch the light on, and see it was only a coil of rope, but your heart will still be pumping like mad. Our bodies react to what we *think* is true.

In 1962, the Kyushi Journal of Medical Science (Japan) reported how the immune systems of Japanese children reacted to their expectations of what was "real." When the children, blindfolded, were told that poison ivy was to be brushed against their arms they produced strong allergic reactions, such as swelling, redness and itching. On the other hand, if they were told that they were being touched by something harmless, these reactions did not appear. Also, the allergic reactions manifested even if they were brushed with some harmless plant, if they had been told it was poison ivy.

When we use affirmations we are making use of this phenomenon that is happening all the time, namely, telling ourselves such and such a thing is so, and feeling and acting on it. The difference is that we deliberately choose a positive viewpoint rather than a negative one. And who is to say which is "real"? It is all a matter of interpretation. As Shakespeare expressed it, "There is nothing either good or bad, but thinking makes it so." (*Hamlet, Act II Scene ii*).

AFFIRMATION TECHNIQUES

1. An affirmation should be short and make a single statement at a time.

2. It should always state the affirmative, rather than deny the negative e.g., *"I am full of courage,"* rather than *"I feel no fear."*

3. It should always be framed in the present, and state that what you want to happen is already the case.

4. An affirmation should be repeated twice, to allow time for it to sink in.

5. The more relaxed you are, the deeper it will sink into the subconscious.

When we use affirmations we are in fact practising auto-suggestion. As in hypnosis, we create another reality for ourselves through the medium of words. It was Emile Coué who discovered the healing power of suggestion at his clinic in Nancy at the beginning of this century. He always insisted that an effort of will was not required—just suspension of disbelief. We now know that this is in fact the case because all effort, all willing, activates the left side of the brain, and it is in fact to the passive, receptive, right side of the brain that affirmations are addressed.

Coué's most famous affirmation, *"Every day, in every way, I am getting better and better,"* is a useful one, for it is so vague that it covers almost everything, and our subconscious will take from it what it needs to hear and apply it to our special needs. In the experience of the author, this affirmation is also a lifeline when one is so far down that to formulate more specific positive statements seems a herculean task. In those moments, just grasp hold of the opening words, *"Every day, in every way"* . . . try to remember the rest of the affirmation—and just go on repeating it, whatever else your mind is telling you, no matter how bad you are feeling. By doing so, you will be reversing the deeper descent into the morass and, gradually, your desperate mood will start to shift, lighten up.

There seems to be some difference of opinion as to how often one should repeat affirmations, whether as often during the day as one remembers, or at times specially set aside to practise them. It could be that by "overdoing" them one is revealing anxiety that they might not really work. It is also possible that one might get bored with them and slip into gabbling them automatically if one does them too often. You could try the following suggestions and see how you get on.

When to Use Affirmations

1. To cancel out a negative programming thought at any time as soon as you become aware of it, merely re-affirm the direct opposite of what you have been telling yourself, e.g., cancel out "I'm feeling exhausted" with, *"I am flowing with radiant energy."*

2. At specific times of the day when you are naturally more relaxed than at others, e.g., on awakening in the morning, just before an afternoon nap, or before falling asleep at night.

3. Before anything that could possibly be considered an ordeal, or something you are apprehensive about.

Examples of Affirmations

All-Purpose Affirmations

I feel stronger with every moment that passes.
With every breath I feel more alive.
There is no limit to how good I can feel.
I feel well, I look well, I am well.
I deserve to be radiantly healthy.

Upon Awakening

Every day, in every way, I am getting better and better.

Before Undergoing Tests

The doctors are amazed at my progress.

Before Taking Treatment or Medication

This treatment is totally successful and feels totally comfortable.
My pills are working wonders—and with no side effects.

After Surgery

The operation is a total success.
Everything is healing as it should.

Before Sleeping

The quality of my life improves, day by day.
When I wake up I shall feel totally refreshed, energised, and well.

For specific ailments you can make up your own affirmations. Here are a few examples:

Anaemia

My blood is rich and replenishes itself daily.

AIDS (see also Part 3)

My immune system is back to full strength again.
I am divinely protected against all infection.

Arthritis

My joints are supple again, and feel smooth and comfortable.

Asthma

I am totally relaxed, breathing fully and freely.

Cancer

My doctors are amazed at my total remission.
My body is healing itself totally.

Heart Trouble

My heart is strong again, and functioning normally.

Taped Affirmations

You can buy pre-recorded "positive thinking" tapes, and
some of these are listed in the Resources appendix. These can
be played at any time, and will re-programme your subconscious whether you are actually listening to them or not. It has
been found, for example, that patients undergoing surgery and
under deep anaesthesia can be affected by the conversation
going on among the surgical team, or by music being played
during the operation. So, you could switch on a tape before
dropping off to sleep—and leave it running. Also, you can
make your own tape of affirmations specifically geared to cancelling out your own special brand of negative thinking, and
add more affirmations to it as you uncover more examples of
depressing things you habitually tell yourself. It has been
found that listening to your own voice is more effective for
re-programming than listening to somebody else's.

Learn to Persevere

My own experience of using affirmations has been that they
do make you feel better, at least temporarily. And they do
make a difference to how you let professional medical staff
approach your body. You will feel more relaxed, for example,
when having blood tests or transfusions if you have programmed yourself for an easy time, than if you are tense and
dreading the needle. Perhaps because your skin and muscles
are more relaxed, or because your calm aura affects the person
working on you, it all goes so much more smoothly.

I remember once having to have a transfusion as I had become very anaemic. I did not do my affirmations and was very jumpy. Each time anyone came near me some disaster happened. The doctor doing the pre-transfusion test kept mumbling that he "could not find the vein"—and when he eventually did, managed to spill blood all over my new trousers. The (normally super-capable) nurse managed to dislodge the cap from the bag as she was setting it up, sending my AB Rhesus Negative group blood splattering over the floor. Incredibly, this happened not once, but twice. It looked like Vietnam all over again. And the more rattled I got, the more clumsy she seemed to get. Eventually, unnerved, she fled and handed me over to another nurse. This is an absolutely true story. And the moral is, don't forget to programme yourself for an easy time.

Do persevere with affirmations, even if the totally opposite reality is staring you in the face day after day and you feel like a liar, as if you are fooling yourself. Think of yourself as a gardener planting seeds. Nurture them, knowing they are there, even though invisible, in the soil of your subconscious mind. Tend them lovingly, and with faith. By and by, the flowers will start to appear. You begin to notice that things seem imperceptibly different in some way, that something is shifting, lightening up. In place of the gloom and misery, nice things start to happen at last. The more you recognise, acknowledge, and express gratitude for these blessings—however small—the thicker and faster they come.

Don't tell others about your affirmations, this is not an ego-trip. Remember that you have called into existence the power of the Universe to support you in your intention of getting well, so gratitude is more appropriate when it does so. Cancel out in a firm but non-aggressive way anything that is said, perhaps by medical staff or well-meaning but unaware friends, which weakens your faith and your resolve. Remember, the agent of healing (after love) is *belief*:

I am grateful for all the blessings I receive daily.

twelve

VISUALISING HEALTH—AND A BRIGHT FUTURE

The power of positive mental images to get the body to heal itself is now beyond question. Experiments carried out in 1984 at the George Washington Medical Centre in Washington D.C. showed how visualisation strengthens the immune system. Not only did it increase the amount of white blood cells, but also the level of a hormone important to the T helper cells called Thymosin-alpha-1. As we have already seen, the success of the Simontons in America with cancer patients using visualisation is spreading more widely, not only to Cancer Help Centres in Britain, but also to the more orthodox medical establishment. Visualisation, for example, is currently being used with AIDS patients at the Middlesex Hospital in London, and the signs are that soon training patients in visualisation may well be offered as part of routine medical treatment.

One of the most dramatic and publicised recoveries following the use of visualisation has been that of Louis Nassaney. Diagnosed to have Kaposi's sarcoma (KS) in May 1983, he took to his bed and stayed there for seven months, getting weaker and weaker, and deeply depressed. Inspired, however, by his father, he decided to drop his victim role and try to get better again. His doctors were suggesting chemotherapy, since gamma interferon treatment was having no effect. Instead, guided by his "metaphysical counsellor," Louise Hay, he embarked on a programme of vitamin therapy, exercise, acupuncture, visualisation, affirmations, deep relaxation and meditation.

Louise taught him to visualise the KS lesion on his thigh as pencil marks. Every night he would create a mental image of himself erasing the lesion with a pencil rubber. He also visualised his helper cells as rabbits, reproducing themselves at a tremendous rate. After four months, the lesion began to fade and in October 1984, a biopsy at the Los Angeles hospital where he had been treated revealed only dead scar tissue. The lesions returned in 1987, but he maintains a positive attitude and remains in good health. His case is non-aggressive. He decided to share his success to encourage other AIDS sufferers, and has been touring the USA spreading a message of hope. Since then, others have been ''going public'' with similar accounts of how they have healed themselves of AIDS— and visualisation has for all of them proved to be one of the main tools for restoring them to health together with changes in lifestyle, diet and mental attitudes.

If visualisation can be so effective in intractable illnesses like cancer and AIDS, it can help anything.

VISUALISATION TECHNIQUE

1. Make sure you will be undisturbed for, say, half an hour. Lie down in a comfortable position you will want to stay in. Relax as deeply as you can for a few minutes. I like to wear a blindfold, but this is optional, as also is putting on some soothing, slow background instrumental music, or environment sounds (see Appendix, page 193).

2. A healing visualisation would normally include three stages:

   a) Seeing your illness in some objectified way.

   b) Seeing it being brought under control by the medication you are receiving and by your own body's defences.

   c) Seeing yourself restored to perfect health.

3. The most important thing is to actually get the feeling in your body that what you are seeing with your mind is really happening. If you have difficulty in creating visual images it does not matter so long as you can get this feeling in your body.

Work with images that come up spontaneously rather than trying to impose them. Use your own images in preference to those suggested by others, ones that have meaning and power for *you*. That said, here are some examples of the types of visualisation you can adapt for yourself.

VISUALISING YOUR ILLNESS

Using biofeedback, it has been found more effective to visualise in symbols than trying to see in your mind's eye the organs of the body, germs or tumours as they are in reality. Symbols that may suggest themselves for pain, for example, could be jagged edges, angry red flames. Tumours could be gnawing animals like rats. The Simontons have much interesting material in chapter 12 of *Getting Well Again* (see Further Reading) that it would be helpful for you to consult. They suggest that the agents of disease (e.g., cancer cells) should always be symbolised in mental imagery as weak and disorganised, rather than, for example, pictured as ants (difficult to get rid of) or crabs (tough shells), stones (hard to disintegrate) or predatory animals (too strong and fierce). Also, they suggest seeing them as grey (a neutral colour) rather than as strong colours like red or black, to help neutralise feelings about cancer. (Carl Simonton, a doctor practising radiotherapy at Fort Worth, Texas, began to suspect that cancer is related to personality, and especially to the suppression of feelings. Though he continued using radiation therapy, he developed a method of improving the patient's attitudes, expectations and ability to express themselves by using affirmations, visualisations, and encouraging them to depict their feelings on paper, etc. His first success in curing a patient of cancer is described in this book on page 25. Since then there have been many more successes, and Simonton's techniques are now used elsewhere.

VISUALISING HEALING

The agents of healing should be seen as stronger and more vigorous than the agents of disease—and overcoming them. How exactly you visualise either is not as important as being clear who are the "goodies" and who are the "baddies"—and making sure the "goodies" always win in the end. You can thus play "cops and robbers," hunter and hunted, knights and dragons—even rival football teams—on your mental video.

See the heroes attacking the villains in any way that feels right to you. See them devouring, routing, mopping up, flushing away until all is left clean and spotless. Penny Brohn mentions one woman cancer patient she knows who uses a vacuum cleaner on her cancer cells, and leaves it running all the time! Here is a visualization which works directly on the immune system.

"Immune System" Visualisation

Focus your attention on your bones. Feel the marrow, nourishing your blood with T and B cells. See these cells as an army on the march through the terrain of your body, or being transported in barges on the bloodstream to the battle area. See the T cells as generals, instructing their officers (B cells) to send their men (antibodies) into battle, and watch these routing and massacring the enemy (germs, malignant cells). After these have all been killed off, see the medics (monocytes) arriving to remove the corpses (the debris of the dead cells).

Thank your army of cells for doing their job of protecting you so well. Have a good look at them. See how strong they are and how many of them there are in proportion to the suppressor cells—just the right ratio. See each cell surrounded

*by a membrane keeping the internal body of each cell intact
and strong, like armour around a knight. See how vigorous
they are, and how vigilant they are, not only of intruders but
also of each other, with whom they communicate clearly and
decisively whenever they perceive a threat to you. Tell them
you love them, and will support them with all the nutrients
they need—and know you have their total loyalty and support.*

"Healing a Part" Visualisations

*Let your attention focus on the part of your body that is in
trouble. It could be a broken limb, an inflamed joint, a wound,
or some internal organ that is affected. Relax as much as you
can and really try to feel the part that is in distress. What
images of it come into your mind? Stay with these mental
pictures for a while until one seems to be the clearest, most
dominant or persistent image—and work with that one.*

*Start to direct loving attention and the intention of healing
to what you can see in your mind's eye. The medium for this
healing energy you direct should be such that it cleanses,
clears up, soothes, conquers or restores order and symmetry
to what you are probably seeing as in some way dirty, dark,
disorganised, disharmonious, jagged or otherwise in a sorry
state. The agent of healing could be a beam of white light, a
jet of clear crystalline water, a paintbrush or a mop (or a
vacuum cleaner!)—anything in fact that has the power to
make clean, purify, restore order, smooth rough edges or clear
up a mess. Persist with your restoration work until it is finished and the part looks in much better shape than when you
started. Remind yourself that at the very least, you are sending
more blood with reinforcements to the part merely by giving
it your attention. Try to stay relaxed rather than forcing. Experiments have shown that one can warm one's hands by focussing attention on them, but not if one concentrates too
fiercely. Here are a few examples, but it is better if you use
images that come up spontaneously.*

Arthritis

*Picture the joint surfaces as pitted. See yourself rubbing them
with some soothing but powerful agent until they are smooth*

again. (This visualisation was successfully used by the Simon-tons' first "cure").

Fractures

See the break, and mend it with whatever materials you need, just as if you were repairing anything else that had broken or split, e.g., with glue, cellotape, etc. Before you leave it, test that it will hold together and leave it to set.

Inflammations

See the inflamed part, perhaps as red and raw, throbbing, swollen. What do you need to apply to cool it down, to soothe it? It could be ice, or you could apply a cooling cream that you know possesses great healing properties ... Rub the cream in gently, feel it penetrating, cooling, soothing away the redness and swelling.

Always finish up a healing visualisation by picturing the part back to normal again or, if you have been working with symbols, images of order, cleanliness, clarity and health.

VISUALISING HEALTH

"Healthy You" Visualisation

Conjure up a picture of yourself in perfect health, perhaps as you were before you became ill, or as you would like to be. How would you look if you were in radiant health right now? Get the feeling in your body. How does it feel to have lots of energy again, to take your health for granted again as you used to? What would you like to be doing now that you are restored to health? See yourself engaging in that activity, in as much detail as possible.

Keep this picture up your sleeve for trotting out in the times when you feel down and your mind may be telling you that you are *never* going to be fighting fit again. Return to this picture of yourself as vibrantly healthy as often as you wish. We grow towards what we think about. Do not return to picturing yourself as ill again—ever.

VISUALISING A BRIGHT FUTURE

It is also therapeutic to have something to look forward to. If we haven't, the life tends to go out of us. We may get apathetic, and depressed. It has been observed as a fact in New York, for example, that terminally ill Jewish patients rarely die immediately before Yom Kippur. This is almost certainly because they are so looking forward to celebrating with their families that they hang on till the fast is over. So, instead of brooding over how gloomy your future looks to you right now (and the lower your energy the more this is likely to be the case), create positive expectations of a bright future for yourself with the following visualisation.

"Goals" Visualisation

Make plans for when you are well again. What would you like to be doing in the future? What haven't you experienced yet that would be a real "turn on" for you? Perhaps a holiday? If so, where would it be? And what would it be like? Who, for example, would you take with you and what do you envisage would be the highlights of the trip? Try to see it in as much detail as possible—and make sure you include yourself in the pictures, naturally healthy and brimming over with energy, enjoyment and enthusiasm. Or perhaps there are other things you still have to do? Perhaps finish that novel (or begin it), start up a business on your own . . . What changes will you make in your life-style when you are back on your feet again? Who will you choose to see more of, and spend less time with? What can you promise yourself that you can really look for-

ward to? In the dark moments remind yourself of how much living you still want to do.

Martin Brofman, diagnosed with terminal throat cancer and given a few months to live by his doctors, promised himself a trip to the Caribbean Club Mediterranée if he survived until the New Year. He survived, and on the holiday ''happened'' to meet a Zen Buddhist who gave him the information he needed to start on the process of healing himself. Fifteen years later he is alive, well and healing others. The following affirmations will help you to feel you have something to look forward to:

My future is bright, healthy, loving, prosperous and SAFE.
Being healthy, happy, loved and with no problems feels totally SAFE.
My life gets better and better with every day that passes.
With every day that passes I feel stronger and more alive.
I look forward to the future with confidence and trust.

thirteen

LOVING YOURSELF MORE—
AND MORE

Love heals. As Louis Nassaney puts it from his own experience: "No one will heal physically if they don't love themselves first." Self-hatred is the most lethal form of negativity we can indulge in. Quite simply, it's a killer.

And yet, unless we have been brought up by enlightened parents and teachers, we have not been taught to love ourselves. On the contrary, we have been indoctrinated against "being selfish," conditioned to feel guilty of narcissism if we catch ourselves admiring our appearance for example, or immodest if we pat ourselves on the back for some achievement or other. We are afraid of being thought egotistical or boastful, of attracting criticism for being "full of ourselves." So we (especially men) tend only to dare to look at ourselves in mirrors when there is nobody else around, and take care to underestimate ourselves and our achievements, for all the world as if putting oneself down were some sort of virtue. We secretly hanker after, yet are terrified of, appearing "special."

And yet we are special, very special. Everybody is. We are magnificent beings, made in the image of God Himself and Herself. Each of us is unique, with a song to sing that has never been sung before on this planet in quite the same way as we sing it. Each of us was brought into existence to contribute a certain quality to the sum total of energy in this world—and the world would be to that extent impoverished if any of us were not here. Which is the same as saying, not only that God/Life/the Universe—The Whole—loves us and wants us to be here, but that we are IT. As Alan Watts the well-known Buddhist teacher once put it:

I am It and you are It,
He is It and she is It;
We are It and they are It,
It is It—and That is That.

When you know who you are, you know who everybody else is. Far from making you "selfish" and quite awful to other people, realising your own magnificence opens your eyes to the magnificence of others. If you respect who you are, how can you not respect those who are made of the same stuff as you? And, since we treat others the way we treat ourselves, the reverse is also true. If I may be allowed a moment of crudity, if you think of yourself as shit you will treat others like shit. And—as above so below— your body will gradually poison itself with toxins to match the mental image you have of yourself.

The importance of a healthy self-image cannot be over-emphasised. If we do not care for ourselves we will not consider ourselves worth caring *for*. We may not nourish ourselves properly, or look after our bodies and make sure we get adequate exercise and rest. We may not accept nourishment offered by others in the way of warmth and intimacy because we are afraid that if we respond and open up they will see what we are really like. All the love in the world may come our way, but unless we, deep down, think we are lovable, it will not reach us. Either we will not let it in, won't trust it, or we won't even see it is there. We won't ask for what we need if we do not think we deserve to get it. We will tend to live our lives "on the outside," as if everybody else had more right to be here than us. And others will always be more OK than us. We will torture ourselves with comparing ourselves with them, and "they" will always be *more* than us: more attractive, successful, clever, popular, outgoing, articulate, and always having a better time than us. By and by, we become a prey to victim consciousness and the acid thoughts that go with it: envy, guilt, resentment, paranoia, and depression. Acid thoughts create acid blood, and in the absence of love, the thymus atrophies even further, bringing down our immune system with it.

It is probably not far wrong to say that, unless you start learning to love yourself, none of the healing techniques described in this book are going to do much good, at least more than temporarily. For you will be contradicting yourself, on the one hand acting as if you were worth healing, yet sabotaging your efforts at a subconscious level by holding on to a mental pattern that tells you that this is not so, that you are not worth healing, would rather not be here. All your dieting, affirming, visualising will be just mechanical, with no heart in it. Self-healing is a function of *love*: of loving your body and wanting it to get well again, of loving life and wanting to be well enough to enjoy it again to the utmost, of loving yourself enough to think you deserve quality and the best there is, of wanting to be well again to enjoy sharing intimacy with those you love.

Be aware that you will probably experience resistance to breaking a lifetime's pattern of self-invalidation when you start practising the exercises in self-love described below. You may feel phoney, unsafe, "tempting the gods" with your arrogance or with sneaking feelings of guilt at being so "immodest." The more your resistance, the more imperative that you break through it, for it is a measure of how deeply ingrained your self-hatred is. *Fake it till you make it.* It could be literally a matter of life and death.

DAILY AFFIRMATIONS

We suggest time should be set aside, at least once daily, for affirming your self-worth, and continued for at least a month. Affirmations should be repeated aloud twice, firmly and with total conviction. Make up your own specifically geared to your own particular brands of self-doubt, the areas in your life where you feel you don't "measure up." Make a tape of your own voice and add to it more self-affirming statements as they suggest themselves to you. Here are some to start off with.

Examples of Affirming Statements

I love and approve of myself totally, every moment.
I am totally lovable, just the way I am.
I am a magnificent, sensitive, loving, creative and valuable being.
Being loved, healthy, successful and happy feels totally SAFE.
Everybody loves me and supports me wherever I go.
I feel safe everywhere, and with all people.
I forgive myself totally for not sufficiently loving myself in the past.
The more I realise my true worth, the more everybody respects me.
I deserve the best of everything, including perfect health.
The more I take care of myself, the more others take care of me.
God wants me to be happy.
I rejoice in my sexuality and enjoy it tremendously.
There is no limit to how good I can feel.
It is my birthright to be totally healthy, happy and fulfilled in everything I do.
I now win all the time.

Louise Hay recommends that one take a mirror and look into one's own eyes and then repeat several times as gently and lovingly as one can: *I really, really love you.* This can be a very powerful exercise. The first time I tried it, my eyes filled with tears and I felt choked. If this happens to you, it is good. You are making a big dent in your conditioning. Keep at it. And if you have some negative "trips" about your body (too fat, too skinny etc, etc.) you could try doing this exercise naked in front of a full length mirror—and love whatever you see.

At first, of course, all this will feel like just "words, words, words." Persevere, and sooner or later you will actually start to FEEL your heart chakra beginning to respond to this reprogramming. Your friends may in fact notice before you do that you seem softer in some way, gentler, more open to them, and somehow more relaxed and calm. They may tell you that they see some quality in your eyes that was not there before—

perhaps because you are beginning to look at them with the same eyes with which you are beginning to look at yourself, more lovingly, less critically, with more acceptance and warmth.

VISUALISATIONS

"Your Perfect Self" Visualisation

Imagine a being standing a few feet away in front of you. Visualise this being as possessing all the ideal qualities you can think of, as perfect as you yourself would like to be. Whatever your highest values, ascribe them to this being: beauty, honesty, courage, humour, grace, awareness, compassion... Keep going through the list of ideal attributes until you can think of no more. The more positive energy you see in this being, the more radiant it becomes. Contemplate this radiant and perfect (and perfectly healthy) being, and know that it is your potential. All these qualities must be in you otherwise you would not be able to recognise them. This high being knows this and, as you contemplate him or her silently, blissfully, you hear the words: I AM YOU AND YOU ARE ME. Your perfect being now moves slowly closer to you... closer and closer until you merge with each other. There is now only YOU. Feel what it is like to be perfect, whole, complete—and radiantly healthy. Enjoy this feeling for as long as you wish— and remember it so that you can recall it whenever you wish.

"Receiving Love" Visualisation

Think of somebody you know who loves you and wants you to be healed. Imagine that this person is standing beside you, wishing you well. Allow yourself to feel this loving energy coming from them. Feel it penetrating your body, enveloping you in soft warmth. Feel too how you love this person and trust they wish you well, and open yourself more and more to the love they want you to receive.

Now imagine this person is joined by another person who also loves you and wants you to be healed. Feel that love as much as you can. Allow it in. Love heals—and you deserve to be healed. Thank that person for wanting you to get well, and feel the love you have for them also.

Continue to gather around you everybody you can think of who you know loves you and wishes you well until you are surrounded by them. Feel the love being beamed at you and allow yourself to open up to it more and more. Now direct that love to the part of your body that most needs healing right now. Love is energy. Feel that energy flowing into the suffering part or system, warming it, cleansing it, making it whole again . . . Bathe in this loving energy, immerse yourself in it, soak it in, surrender to it. Enjoy the bliss for as long as you want, then come back into yourself. Thank your friends for their love and tell them you love them as well. Then relax for a while, as you would after a massage, instead of scattering the energy that has built up. This visualisation has the effect of massaging the thymus.

(This visualisation is based on one of Martin Brofman's. It is available on tape and details of this and others and how to get hold of them are given in the Resources appendix.)

EXPRESS YOUR FEELINGS

One of the most moving experiences of my life happened while I was researching this book. I had signed up for a weekend group with a well-known healer, hoping to learn more about this endlessly fascinating subject. Some of the participants in the group were trainee healers themselves, but others were quite ill, some with AIDS or cancer.

On the last day of the group, the leader eventually got round to one of the women with whom she had not yet worked, and who had made herself almost invisible the whole weekend. She had asked no questions, volunteered no information about herself apart from the fact that she had breast cancer, kept very much to herself during breaks. She was a tiny woman, of indeterminate age and very subdued. She looked visibly nervous when the group leader stopped in front of her and said cheerfully, "Now it's your turn. Can you tell us a bit about yourself, why you came to this weekend, maybe?" Silence. The woman sat stiffly, shoulders hunched, looking at the floor.

The healer got down to her level, squatting on her haunches and placing both hands on the woman's knees. Softly, she asked, "Was it because you want to be healed?" Still silence. "Can you look at me?" was the next question, asked quietly and with tremendous gentleness. The woman looked up. "Do you want to be healed?" The woman nodded in reply.

"So, tell me that. Tell me you want to be healed," said the healer. Hesitantly, after what seemed an age, the woman finally spoke, in a voice so low we all leaned forward on our chairs to catch her faint reply "Yes."

"No!," said the group leader, unexpectedly tough. "I'm not going to let you get away with that. I want to hear you say it. Yes what?"

"Yes . . . I want to be healed," the woman managed to say.

"Great! I know it was hard for you to say that. Well done. I get a strong impression that it's hard for you to say what you want. Is that accurate?" Another nod. "So let's make a start now in breaking that habit. I would like you to tell me what else you want for yourself. Will you do that?" Silence. You could have heard a pin drop. The woman just couldn't do it. The words would not come out. There was not a dry eye in the room as we all resonated with the woman's struggle with the conditioning we have all been subjected to against daring to ask for what we want.

The group leader eventually got her to repeat some phrases after her, like "I want to get well," "I want to be happy" and tried to get her to see the urgency for her healing of speaking up for herself for a change. Eventually, standing up, she said to the woman with deep feeling. "You really do have to start asking for what you want. For you, it's a matter of life and death."

Every time we do not risk asking for what we need we die

a little. Each time we suppress a feeling because we "shouldn't" feel this way we deaden ourselves more. And each time we say "yes" when we really mean "no" we stop ourselves flowing with our energy, dry up a little more, become less authentic and real. We are here to feel and to express ourselves. It is why we have a body at all. Energy has to go somewhere, and the energy generated by feeling and emotion, if not expressed in some way in the outer world, turns in upon ourselves and goes sour. The link between unexpressed feelings and illnesses, from the common cold to cancer, is now well known. As we have seen, it is the "nice" person who is most likely to develop cancer—and the "difficult" patient who is most likely to survive it.

And yet from a very early age we have been conditioned to be nice, and not to be difficult. Unless we have been very fortunate, we have been educated, not for authenticity but for conformity. We were rewarded—and still are— when we told people what they wanted to hear rather than what we really felt. We learned that the love given to us was conditional—on pleasing, on expressing only the "good" parts of us, on meeting expectations. To ask directly for what we wanted was risky; we might not get it, it might be disapproved of, we might be being selfish. So in the process of growing up, in order to feel loved, we all developed two subpersonalities that have had a stranglehold on us ever since: a Pleaser and a Controller. Between them, these two parts of us straitjacket the other parts of us, inhibiting our freedom of expression, making us always look over our shoulder to make sure it's OK with others before we please ourselves, trying to live up to expectations as to how we "should" be—and suppressing any feelings or desires that don't "fit" that image.

Our culture is so heavily loaded on rewarding achievement that many of us develop other subpersonalities that are obsessively goal orientated, the "Workaholic," for example, and the "Perfectionist." Between them, these two "keep us on the go," make sure we "come up to scratch," and drive us relentlessly. They are responsible for causing more coronaries than anything else, for the stress we put on ourselves is always more lethal than anything that comes at us from the outside. The curious thing is that we will kill ourselves to get love and

to feel OK by attempting to live up to what we are not. And
the silliest thing is that it never works: for, deep down, we
know that what people are approving of is only the image we
are presenting to please, not the real us. So the Child inside
us remains perpetually unsatisfied, longing to be loved for itself, unconditionally, just as it is, with all its vulnerability, lack
of sophistication and, yes, naughtiness.

Changing Your Attitude to Your Needs

Being ill has its advantages. Use them. In fact, your Inner
Child may have brought you to your sickbed precisely in order
to enjoy some of these advantages that you would not allow
it when you were well. What are these advantages? Well, the
main one is that people have fewer expectations of you. You
don't have to go to work, be a responsible citizen, always be
polite even when you are bored to death, or put other people's
preferences before your own. I am not suggesting that you
become a pain in the neck and a burden to everybody around
you. I am simply suggesting that, perhaps for the first time in
your life, you give yourself permission to *please yourself first*
and refrain from doing anything you don't feel like doing.

This may be hard at first, for we are not prepared for following our own rhythms, flowing with our energy, and staying
in touch with our own needs as they surface into consciousness
from moment to moment. If this sounds rather like becoming
a child again, it is. However, it is not about being childish in
the sense of throwing tantrums, but about regaining the freshness and spontaneity of the Child within you and nourishing
it. And since your Inner Child has always been the most authentic and alive part of you—perhaps in spite of all your
attempts to suppress it and keep it hidden—in nourishing it
you will be helping to bring yourself back to life at a very
deep level. Remember that children are also playful: it was
nurturing this aspect of his Inner Child that enabled Norman
Cousins to heal himself of an "incurable" illness (see page
16).

Our Inner Child is also vulnerable, and needs holding and
to feel safe. Allow yourself to ask for support, to share your

vulnerability, and perhaps your panic, too. You don't need a professional counsellor, just somebody whom you trust who can listen to you and be there. Touching is important too. Often, when you are feeling down, needy, and not knowing what it is you need, a hug does wonders. Risk asking for one.

The more seriously ill you are, the more you need to allow yourself to be more authentic, to say what you mean and mean what you say, to ask for what you want—and to say what you do not want. The time is past for pretending to be who you are not. This may be hard on people close to you who are accustomed to casting you in a certain role. But then again it could also be a relief and bring you closer.

One of the things that becomes easier to say when it is possible that you may not be around for much longer is "I love you." As we enter a new phase in our relationship to AIDS—from judgement and paranoia to understanding and compassion—stories are beginning to emerge of how parents, learning for the first time of their son's homosexuality, have rallied beautifully in support and allowed him to die feeling perhaps for the first time, seen, loved and accepted for who he is.

We have already suggested that "leading a double life" is deleterious for the immune system. In a sense, to a greater or lesser degree, we all of us lead double lives, for few of us are honest enough, courageous or outrageous enough, and, yes, rich enough, to be ourselves all the time.

It may not be so important to *get* what you want as to say what you want. The first may not always be possible, but the second always is. And speaking up for yourself is an expression of your own self-esteem and self-respect. Whether or not you get your own way is not as important as the statement you are making:

> *Here I am.*
> *I have as much right to be here as anybody else.*
> *I matter.*

fourteen

LISTENING TO YOUR INNER SELF

There are no accidents and it is no accident you have been ill. Illness (like everything else) can be a learning experience. It has lessons to teach us, and it is possible that the reason why we become ill at all is because this is the only way we can learn what we need to learn. What these lessons mean to you is a highly personal affair: only you are in a position to work them out. How you do this is very much centred on listening to yourself—or rather your selves—and asking for guidance.

What sort of lessons does illness teach us? Basically, it teaches us about balance and change, how we have been living out of balance and what changes we need to make in our life-styles and mental patterns in order to restore that balance. Below, we discuss some of the things you might discover about yourself and why you became ill. It becomes clear when you start asking yourself these questions: "What does this illness mean?" "Why has it come at this time in my life?," "Why has it taken this form?," and, most relevant of all, "What do I need to do to heal myself?"

One of the things that being ill certainly does for us is give us time to reflect on what we are doing with our lives. Take advantage of this time, this breathing-space amid the hurly-burly and rush of "trying to keep it all together." Perhaps this is exactly what you needed to get back in contact with your self, to become aware of your deeper needs and how you may have kept yourself too busy to even be aware of them, let alone fill them. And remember that it is not enough just to smash your symptoms with chemotherapy or surgery. Unless you make the necessary changes in the ways you think, feel and act, you may merely create the illness again, perhaps in another part of the body.

Here is a technique you might find useful in this process of tuning into what your illness may really be about and what sort of patterns you might need to change in order to get well again. You don't have to do it all in one go, but as it feels right.

MEDITATIONS ON THE CHAKRAS

Each of the seven chakras is a channel for energies we use to handle the situations that come up in specific areas of our lives (refer to the chart on page 34). Any area which we are not handling successfully or in which we are experiencing worry and stress will affect the flow of energy through that particular chakra, which will result in imbalance in the body. If we give ourselves time and space to look at these different areas of our lives in turn, to reconsider the past experiences in each from which we have distilled the way we think and feel now, we can pinpoint the ways in which we put ourselves under stress, e.g., with impossible expectations of ourselves, with double binds, with resistance to accepting our needs, etc. Important clues will be provided by the sort of symptoms that you have produced in your body and where, for these symptoms are often metaphors on the physical plane for where we are stuck on a psychic level in rigid mental patterns. If you can decipher the message of these symptoms—and act on the information they are trying to give you by letting go of self-limiting ideas—they will have served their purpose and hopefully will disappear back into the nothingness from which they came. Meditation means giving relaxed attention, not "concentrating" or thinking, but using your intuition and allowing the answers to come from the part of you in the Unconscious that always knows what your truth is.

Meditation on the chakras is a convenient way of looking systematically at significant areas of your life where unbalanced or blocked energy may have contributed to your illness. Remember, *dissolving patterns dissolves disease.*

First Chakra: Your Relationship to Survival, the Earth, the Mother

When you start to reflect on where you are "at" in the basic business of survival on this planet, and whether this has always been hard for you or "you have it made," you may get in touch with a constant source of stress that perhaps was only hitherto dimly felt, and was perhaps taken for granted. Do you worry about having enough money to live on? Do you feel supported by your environment and trust that you will always have enough? Or do you always feel vaguely unsafe, perhaps used to living from hand to mouth, constantly coping with crisis situations—or fearing them? Does the world feel safe, or more like a jungle? Before you fell ill, did you have any vague feelings that it was all becoming too hard, that you would like to give up and be cared for for a change?

What is your relationship with Nature and Mother Earth? Do you feel grounded? Do you make regular contact with Nature, even if it's only going for walks in the park and enjoying the flowers, and allowing it to nourish your inner self? Or do you live all the time in a concrete jungle, never feeling the grass beneath your feet, never thinking to give yourself the experience of enjoying the beauty of a sunset, a starry or full moon night, or a spectacular landscape?

How is (was) your relationship with your mother? Did you feel supported emotionally by her when you were a child? Did you experience her as strong and there for you, or did she seem so fragile and vulnerable that you were afraid of draining her, by being naughty, for example, or making demands? Do you have "unfinished business" with her, resentments or guilt, things that have never been expressed between you that perhaps needed to be? Do (or did you) feel *seen* by her, and loved for who you are rather than what she wanted you to be? How easy was it to break away from her apron-strings without feeling responsible for her or guilty?

Allow yourself to feel what is true for you in this very basic area of survival, of keeping body and soul together. If you get in touch with sources of stress, feelings for example of anxiety or insecurity, try to pinpoint exactly what these are about—and use affirmations to unblock the energy. Here are a few examples:

Affirmations

I am not my mother. I do not have her thoughts and feelings.
I love my mother, and I am not responsible for her happiness.
I forgive my mother for all the ways I mistakenly thought she hurt me.
I feel safe everywhere.
I relax and trust the environment to support me.
I have enough. I shall always have enough.
My life gets easier and easier every day.
I always get what I need, when I need it.

Changes That Might Suggest Themselves for When You Are Well

• Working on your relationship with your mother.

• Giving more attention to becoming financially secure.

• Becoming aware of the needs for security of your Inner Child—and taking more care to make it feel safe in any way you can, for example, by taking fewer risks, not exposing it to scary situations.

• Strengthening your connection with Nature and the Earth.

• Grounding yourself more, for example, by taking more exercise, or learning yoga or tai-chi ("meditation in action"—slow movements performed with total awareness).

• Slowing down, and staying in the present rather than future-tripping; "losing your mind and coming to your senses."

- Being more *physical*, being more aware of your body and looking after it better.

- Relaxing and enjoying yourself more rather than worrying so much.

"Grounding" Visualisation

Sit in a chair with your back straight but relaxed, and your feet uncrossed, soles flat on the floor. Close your eyes, take a few deep breaths, and focus on the very base of your spinal cord. Visualise your spinal cord slowly lengthening downwards, dividing into two branches or roots that pass slowly down both legs. Feel your feet planted firmly on the floor as the roots pass through them and down into the earth. Deeper and deeper they go, making you feel "rooted," "grounded," solid and securely based . . . Enjoy this safe feeling for a while as you watch the main roots, putting out secondary roots, spreading out under the earth . . . Now feel the energy from the Earth spreading up slowly through those roots into the soles of your feet. Imagine that this energy is molten red, like lava from a volcano. Feel it warming you as it passes up your legs and the two "branches" join up again at the base of your spine.

Stay with this feeling of being "rooted" in the ground and nourished by Mother Earth, and enjoy how "solid" and safe you feel.

Second Chakra: Your Relationship to Sex and Sensuality

This second chakra is very much to do with how you relate to the earthier energies that come through you (especially sexual energy), what you do with your "gut feelings" about yourself and other people, how you feel about your body and bodily functions, how fully you allow yourself to enjoy the pleasure these can bring.

Sex is an area of great confusion for many people. Understandably so, for we are given so many double messages about it, not only in the process of growing up (assuming it is even mentioned at all and is not a totally taboo subject in the family circle), but in the hypes with which we are bombarded daily by the media, films and novels. The puritanical strain in the Judeo-Christian tradition, its insistence on linking human sexuality exclusively to procreation (perpetuated in the Roman Catholic prohibition of "artificial" contraception) makes sinners out of most heterosexuals and invalidates all homosexuals. For the latter particularly, and women experiencing problems of dependence in relationships, this second chakra is an area which will probably need to be worked on.

Consider your sex life so far. What are your feelings about it? Has it been on the whole satisfying and enriching—or a series of disasters? What are your preferences? Do you have any negative feelings about sex, such as doubts about the adequacy of your performance, or guilt at promiscuity—or at doing it at all? When you think of your partners so far, what do you feel about them? What were they really to you and at what level of intimacy and honesty did you allow yourself to relate to them? How attractive do you rate yourself as a sexual partner? How do you feel about your body and your bodily functions? How afraid are you of growing older and loosing your desirability as a sexual partner?

How much freedom do you allow yourself sexually? Do you please yourself, or are you primarily concerned that your partner feels satisfied? How trapped in "male" and "female" roles are you, or in manipulative games?

If you have been promiscuous, what was that about? Did it get you what you needed or did you end up lonelier than before the encounter? Which needs do you try to satisfy through sex? Does it work? If not, why do you think this is so? If you are in a monogamous relationship, how satisfied are you with it? If you are not in such a relationship, why do you think this is so?

How are you with sensuality and enjoyment? Do you enjoy your body and your senses, or do you have a nagging feeling of guilt whenever you are having a good time? When work is over, and you have free time, is it hard for you to find ways to occupy yourself pleasurably? Or is the reverse true, namely that if you are not out on the town every night you feel bored and restless? How do you feel about spending time alone with yourself?

You may find that your balance in this chakra needs correcting in that either you don't validate your own sexuality and don't give yourself permission to express it in ways fulfilling to you, or you go "over the top" and make it the centre of your life, probably because you have too much invested in it. More than perhaps in any other area of one's life, one has above all to be *discriminating* in the sexual arena. The penalties for unawareness and confusion can be dire, and never more so than today.

Try some of the following affirmations to see whether they "fit" you. You will know if you have "hit a block" by feeling a resistance to saying them or a subtle resonance in your body.

Affirmations on Sexuality

I am free to express my sexuality as I choose.

I enjoy my sexuality tremendously.

It is OK to enjoy myself.

I no longer settle for what I can get, but only for what I want.

Being attractive, loved, and physically close feels totally SAFE.

I forgive all those who tried to make me feel guilty about sex and my body.

I care for myself enough not to expose myself to physical risks or emotional damage.

If there's no feeling in it, I don't want it any more.

The more I enjoy myself, the more alive I feel.

God wants me to enjoy myself.

The happier I am, the happier people are around me.

I am an interesting, attractive, sensitive and feeling person.

I didn't fail in that relationship—I grew out of it.

My lovers have been my teachers and I am grateful to them.

I have learned from my experiences, even if sometimes they were painful.

I respect myself enough to say "yes" only when I mean it.

I am not interested in relating to anybody who does not respect me as much as I respect myself.

I value myself enough to settle only for the best.
I enjoy my own company, and so do others.

Things You Might Find You Have to Work On

• Sexual guilt.

• Unfinished business with former lovers.

• Forgiving yourself e.g., for promiscuity, for your treatment of another.

• Grief or resentment at having been left for another.

• Whether or not to stay in a current relationship.

• Issues of dependence on your partner.

• Low self-image.

• How to "loosen up" and enjoy yourself more.

"Confronting the Guilt-Mongers" Visualisation

Relax and close your eyes. Focus your attention on the area just above your genitals, a few inches below your navel.

Imagine yourself sitting at a desk in a room where you feel totally on your own territory and safe. Let your mind wander back to your childhood and try to remember what messages were given to you about your body and your sexuality and by whom. Who, for example, ever punished or threatened to punish you for sexual activity of any kind? From whom did you hear messages that you interpreted as meaning that sex, you, or your body were bad?

One by one, summon each of these people into your presence. See them standing before you. Remind them of the incident and how it affected you. Wait for their response. Try to understand the place they were coming from and the effects on them of their own conditioning about sex. When you have heard them out, tell them you disagree with their views and deliver a little lecture about what your sexuality means to you. Be positive. Totally validate your freedom to be a sexual being in the way that is most natural for you. Finish up by telling them you forgive them for passing their hang-ups on to you when you were too young to recognise a hang-up when you saw one—and dismiss them.

Third Chakra: Your Relationship to Power

For many people, "power" is a dirty word. It has the connotations of controlling and manipulating others, of egoism and exploitation. We often are afraid to own our own power. Indeed, we fear it or the antagonism of others if we challenge their attempts to manipulate, invalidate or otherwise not respect our space or who we are. We have been conditioned to be "nice" and to please, rather than to be authentic, clear and honest in our communications, "upfront." Our overdeveloped "Pleaser" never lets us feel that we matter as much as other people, or that it's OK to please ourselves. It makes us apologetic, self-effacing, unable to defend ourselves under attack, and, ultimately, victims. It is understandable that victim-consciousness is mirrored in the body by an impaired immune system, for if we feel defenceless on a psychic plane this will be mirrored in depressed activity by the defenders within—the T and B cells.

The sorts of things that might come up for you here are issues of control, ambition, success and achievement, or lack of it in your life, feeling able to confront and stand your ground—or being a "pushover," feeling confident, in charge of your life and able to cope, or feeling inferior to others and a victim. Imbalance in the third chakra is very common in our materialistic, success-orientated and competitive society, in which many people's sense of their self-worth is measured by their economic status and possession of the things that are the symbols of that status. Striving continuously to amass more— or falling behind in the rat-race—is stressful. The experience of frustration and disappointment, failure to cope, loss of economic or personal power, for example, through redundancy or enforced retirement are very often precipitating factors in illness.

Questions to Ask Yourself

The following questions will help you understand why you became ill:

- What stresses was I under immediately before I fell ill?

- What choices did I make which allowed this stress to build up so much?

- What fuels my Workaholic and Perfectionist sub-personalities, in other words why do I drive myself so hard?

- What do I feel I need to prove?

- What does it profit a man (or a woman) if they gain the whole world and lose their health?

- Who and what have power over me?

- How, exactly, do I give my power away?

- Am I able to say "No" and mean it?

- What am I addicted to, e.g., work, being in control, being right, manipulating my energy through drugs? Why do I need these?

- How do I relate to authority e.g., do I need it, am I oppressed by it?

Changing Negative Patterns

It really is important not to blame yourself when you get insight into a self-defeating or self-destructive pattern. Rather, congratulate yourself for having uncovered a little saboteur of your happiness and wellbeing of whose existence you have hitherto been unaware but can now bring out into the light of consciousness and challenge. These are only ideas, attitudes: they can be changed, for example by using affirmations. And each time you are honest enough to take responsibility for having taken on board a limiting pattern of thought or behaviour you *ipso facto* dis-identify with it and take back your power to choose no longer to think or act slavishly in the same old way. Freedom is not cheap; it has to be worked for. But once you get to see how much your life and experience changes for the better when you drop ideas that no longer work for you, it becomes a joy "lightening up" by getting rid of what is, at best, excess luggage, at worst, mere garbage. Some of the things you might have to work on might include:

- Reviewing your priorities and what you really want out of life.

- Understanding your addictions and what drives you.

- Dropping your more stressful attachments.

- Relieving the pressures on you, for example, by delegating, restructuring work schedules, taking early retirement or at least time off.

- Taking back your power to live the way *you* want to live.

- Refusing to be a victim any longer.

- Realising you always have choice—and exercising it.

- Choosing the *experience* of quality of life rather than the symbols of it.

Affirmations to Cancel Out the Negative

When you have achieved some clarity about what you need to change in your assumptions or life-style, "clinch" it by making a statement about how you want to be from now on. Cancel out any negative pattern by composing an affirmation that states the direct opposite. Carry it around with you during the day like a mantra. Repeat it often. Feel the energy that goes with it in your body. Act as if you already are this sort of person. *Fake it till you make it*—and you will. Here are some affirmations which might fit your particular needs:

I do not have to try so hard. I have enough. I am enough.
I am master of my own life and my own authority.
No person and no thing has power over me.
I am free to live in any way I choose.

I am not here to meet anybody's expectations.
It's OK for me to relax and take time off.
I have the courage and strength to stand up for myself.
From now on I don't do anything I don't want to do.

"Perfect Life-style" Visualisation

Visualisation works because it makes use of the mechanism by which our bodies obediently get to work to manifest, to make a reality of whatever pictures are being projected on our mind-screens. Whether these pictures are "real" or fantasy is irrelevant, for the body cannot distinguish. In addition, our mental pictures set up vibrations which are broadcast to our "outer body" (the Universe) and attract the sort of experiences which match the pictures. To visualise is therefore a deliberate act of creation arising out of your love and respect for yourself and your power to choose to give yourself good or bad experiences. It makes use of the illogical yet none the less real psychological "law of effect" which states; "Produce the effect and the cause will follow." In other words, choose to be happy first, and soon reasons for you to be happy will appear around you. Try this visualisation:

Focus your attention on your solar plexus, and breathe into it. Start to tune in, at a "gut level," to what you really want for yourself. At first the images that come up may be things, possessions, status. What is their meaning for you? How would possessing them make you feel good? What are they symbols for? What is lacking in your life and how have you been trying to fill this lack? Has it worked—or have you merely exhausted yourself by going for the symbol and not the real experience? Allow yourself to really feel the difference between these two.

Visualise yourself as already having a totally satisfying life-style, feeling completely fulfilled and happy. See it in as much detail as possible. How are you living, where and with whom? How do you spend your day? What things particularly give you pleasure? (Allow yourself to be surprised by whatever wants to come into your consciousness that perhaps you did not expect). Be aware of any feelings of discomfort at giving yourself an easy time for a change, and ask yourself what that is about. Who have you been trying to please? Whose expectations of you have you been trying to live up to? How does it feel to please yourself for a change and live according to the way you choose, rather than what you have been taught you should choose?

Finally, what changes and choices would you have to make in your present lifestyle for you to get this new quality into your life? Visualise yourself making these changes and choices, and the problems and resistance you might have to encounter. Are you willing to do this?

Fourth Chakra: Your Perceptions of Loving and Being Loved

If any chakra can be said to be more important than any other and certainly for your healing, it is this one. We have seen in Part 1 how the heart chakra is linked closely with the thymus that controls the immune system and how loss of love is the worst form of stress a human being can be subjected to. In one sense also, the heart chakra is the mediator between all the other chakras, being the mid-point between them. In other words, if your heart chakra is closed, your other chakras are bound to be in a state of imbalance. You will see the world as a jungle and never feel secure in it (first chakra), find yourself continually bruised in loveless sexual encounters (second chakra), and try to fill the emptiness inside with things and possessions and compensate for your sense of unlovability with the pursuit of power and status (third chakra). Lacking self-worth, distrustful of others, you will tend to hesitate before you express yourself spontaneously for fear of criticism, and you may stifle your creativity because you feel you have nothing of value to offer (fifth chakra). And the higher levels of consciousness will be barred to you (sixth and seventh chakras), as your awareness of what life is about and your relationship to the Whole will be distorted by the fact that you are not able to tune into the wavelength of love that is the deepest reality in the Universe and holds it all together.

Questions to Ask Yourself

The following questions will show if you need to work at the heart chakra. Basically, these questions will be about your image of yourself as a lovable human being or not, about vulnerability and whether you tolerate and allow it in yourself and others, about your Inner Child and its needs and whether you have been or are sensitive to it and whether you have nurtured it. Once again, don't be hard on yourself if you discover just how blocked you may be from giving and receiving tenderness and love. Maybe you just didn't receive enough of it early on in your life to learn how beautiful it is. Or perhaps you are more sensitive than you thought and needed to protect yourself by closing off, by not feeling safe enough to let your vulnerability show. And, as well as not blaming yourself for doing what you needed perhaps to do *then*, don't blame your parents either. They did the best they knew how, given their own hangups. And they had parents too. Here are a few questions to start you off:

- Did you experience any form of loss before getting ill?

- Deep down, do you feel you are lovable, just for being who you are?

- If not, why not? How are you different from the rest of the human race?

- Where do you think this idea came from?

- Do you feel you have to be perfect before anyone will love you?

- If so, what is this "perfection" and how would you have to change?

- Who would you be trying to please by being "perfect"?

- What, if any, are the feelings that are most painful for you to experience or acknowledge to yourself?

- What is your fear of what might happen if you do?

- Which elements of yourself make you ashamed, or make you think others would see them as unacceptable if you revealed them?

- Who, or which experiences in the past, taught you to be ashamed of these parts of you?

- How much intimacy have you been able to tolerate in your life?

- Which types of people are you afraid of, and why?

- How could they hurt you?

- How do you react when you feel hurt?

- In what ways have you been avoiding getting too close to people?

- What are your stratagems for keeping people at a safe distance?

- Which resentments are you still hanging on to?

- Who in your life can you not forgive?

- What have you not forgiven yourself for?

Negative Patterns You Might Need to Work On

We have seen how forgiveness and healing are inextricably linked in terms of energy, as indeed they were in the miracles of Jesus. Unwillingness to forgive (including oneself) and holding on to guilt and resentment can be quite lethal. If you want to get well you must make it a top priority to check out what negative habits of thinking about yourself and others you may be holding on to—and release them. Not for any moralistic reason, but for your own healing.

Remember too that any judgement we make of others diminishes *us* as well as them. What we are saying in fact (whatever the judgement happens to be) is "I am not big enough, tolerant enough, loving enough, to accept this part of reality, I cannot allow myself this particular choice of how to be, so cannot allow it in you either." Not only do our judgements make us contract and block the free flow of energy in us and our relationships, but they attract more of the unwelcome en-

ergy into our personal orbits. Whatever we resist, persists—
until we allow it just to *be*. We don't have to like it (or, even
less, become it). But the psychic law is that all energies have
to be *honoured* for them not to take their revenge for our
disownment of them. (Read *Who's Pulling Your Strings?*—
see Further Reading—for a fuller explanation of this topic.)
You may need to work on:

• Self-hatred.

• Guilt.

• Holding on to resentments.

• Living in the past.

• Unwillingness to forgive—including forgiving yourself.

• Intolerance of others, prejudice and judgementalism.

• Expectations of being ''perfect'' of yourself and others.

• Acknowledging your need for love, being seen, heard and
  held, and for respect and intimacy.

• How you stop yourself experiencing these in your life.

• Inability to receive from others.

• Fear of vulnerability, of being out of control.

• Fear of being swamped by feelings you can't handle.

For suitable affirmations consult chapter 13 Loving Yourself
More—and More (see pages 128–137) and look at Metta Visualisation (pages 107–108) and ''Receiving Love'' Visualisation (pages 132–133).

Fifth Chakra: Self-expression, Communication, Choice, and Creativity

Signs that you need to work on this chakra are feelings of
being ''in a rut,'' trapped by stale routine, discontent and rest-

lessness with things as they are, not being in touch with your own creativity or its wellsprings drying up on you, a sense of not being real or true to yourself, not "really living." This chakra is very much that of flowing manifestation, of spontaneity and authenticity, and of expressing who we are in the world and communicating our true feelings and reality to others.

Life is about change and the emergence of ever-new forms, the manifestation of the potential and the as yet unmanifest, of cycles of growth from seed to embryo, to flowering and bearing fruit. To stay truly alive (and well) one has to risk continually moving on, allowing the new, dropping the known and safe for what is wanting to be born in us. One wonders just how often we need to create illness in our bodies in order to force us out of a rut, a job that perhaps we have stayed in for too long, or a relationship that has "died" on us but which we cling to out of fear—of hurting the other, of ending up alone, of generally falling flat on our faces.

Living continuously with indecision or unresolved conflict, or in an environment where it is not safe for some reason to be oneself, transparent, spontaneous, honest, is, from the point of view of our health, asking for trouble. Remember the "cancer profiles" (see page xvii–xviii), and their recurring theme of inability or unwillingness to express feelings. Remember the connection that is being made between having to hide in the closet and AIDS. And, on a less drastic level, how you used to very conveniently develop a cold, a fever or a tummyache when you hadn't done your homework and wanted to get out of going to school.

Questions to Ask Yourself

The following questions will reveal if you have problems in the fifth chakra:

• In which area(s) of my life do I feel "in a rut"?

• What keeps me in this rut?

• What would have to happen for me to move out of it?

• What would I have to give up?

• Am I willing to do this, to risk making changes?

• In what ways am I not allowing myself to express more of me?

• What do I fear might happen if I did?

• What are the ideas and mental patterns that limit me and keep me trapped?

• In what ways do I continue to cling on to the past?

• How could I be more free to be who I am?

• To what extent am I controlled by my Pleaser and Controller (i.e., my need to censor what I say and do lest others don't like it or I land myself in trouble?)

• Who am I trying to please?

• Why does expressing freely who I am feel threatening?

Confidence-Building Affirmations

It's OK to be who I am—and to express it.
Being myself at all times feels totally safe.
The more I express myself, the happier I feel.
It is my birthright to live my life in any way I choose.
I am not here to meet others' expectations.
To know me is to love me.
It's OK to ask for what I want—and to get it.
I flow with my energy—all the time.
I trust and follow my "gut feelings" at all times.
I acknowledge and support my feelings—whatever they are.
I have the courage and strength to make the changes that need to be made.
If people cannot accept any part of me, that shows their own limitations.
I trust my preferences to show me where my true vocation lies.
I trust the Universe will always support me if I follow my heart.

I no longer limit myself, the sky's the limit.
I am always free to choose how I want to live.

"Total Freedom" Visualisation

Lie down, close your eyes, perhaps put on a relaxing tape of instrumental music that you like. Focus your attention on your throat area.

Now have a fantasy of what it would be like to feel totally free, flowing, enjoying, feeling free to think, say, feel and do whatever you like. No expectations, no demands, just moving from moment to moment according to your own rhythm, flowing with your own energy where it wants to take you. Feel any resistance that may come up about being "selfish." Tell yourself that rather, you are being "self-centred," centred in yourself, rather than dependent on anyone or anything outside yourself to "make" you happy, that you are taking charge of your own life rather than playing the weak, dependent, victim—and having to manipulate and control others to get what you need.

Feel the feeling of fulfilment and freedom that maybe you have not experienced since you were very small. Having this fantasy, you are in fact energising the Child within you, especially in its playful and magical aspects, that you may have been suppressing for years. Allow him or her out now to play. What are the images that come on to your mind screen? What are the symbols of freedom for you? For me a powerful one has always been swimming naked in a warm sea, floating on my back, totally relaxed and contented, screwing up my eyes against the hot sunshine, hearing the seabirds (another symbol of freedom) wheeling and crying overhead . . . Get the feeling in your body of what is left when the (literally) trappings of civilisation are allowed to slough away. How does it feel to be "natural" again, like a child, directly experiencing moment to moment what it means to be alive, real, enjoying . . . ?

Now come back to your "real" life and compare the way you feel most of the time with your fantasy of freedom. Where are the areas in which you do not feel free? Why is this? What exactly are the constraints upon you? What changes would

*you have to make to feel more free in this area of your life?
What are the limiting ideas that have stopped you making
these changes hitherto? What is your choice: to make changes
(perhaps gradually, one at a time) or to leave things as they
are? Whichever you decide, remember—you chose it. That is
your freedom.*

Sixth Chakra: Your Relationship to Your Intuition

You will have been using your intuition already trying to get
insight (which literally means seeing into) into what patterns
you need to change and how you have been limiting yourself.
The more you trust your intuition, the more it develops, rather
like a muscle that you exercise regularly. It is possible that if
you had listened to it more, trusted it and acted on it, you
might have avoided falling ill, for messages from our Unconscious are constantly trying to get through to us via this
chakra. For example, you may have had vague feelings that
all was not well with your health, that you were "going down
with something." I remember once talking to a man who was
recovering from a coronary and hearing him say, "I knew that
I was pushing myself too hard. Something inside me was telling me 'Ease up.' " But he didn't. Vital messages will often
try to come through to us via our dreams.

Intuition is our direct line to the Unconscious. It is a function of the right side of the brain rather than the left, so it is
a feeling rather than a thinking or verbal phenomenon—passive, more like a listening rather than an active doing. It is
therefore yin, a "female" part of us (whatever our gender)
that is very sensitive and feeling and needs to be protected
and supported by the "male" side of us which is capable of
action in the outer world. In other words, when we let our
intuition guide us, and act on the basis of our feeling about
the reality behind appearances, i.e., trust our "hunches," we
won't go far wrong.

This is very true of the healing process. At some level we
always know what is right for us, even though others (or our
minds) are telling us something else. We need however, to
cultivate the ability to listen to the subtle messages, otherwise

we will not hear them. In order to hear the "still, small voice" of our Inner Wisdom, we ourselves need to be still, receptive, wanting to know rather than thinking we know already. This is what meditation is about.

Try asking the part of you that *knows* the following questions:

• What is the message of my illness?

• Why has it come at this time in my life?

• What are the lessons I have to learn from it?

• Why, if at all, did I need this illness?

• In what ways did I help to create it?

• What "payoffs" am I getting from being ill, right now?

• What do I need to do to heal myself?

Ask with confidence that you will get the answers. Maybe they will not come immediately and maybe not in the form you expected. There is a saying in the East "When the disciple is ready, the Guru appears." This means roughly the same as the words of Jesus, "Ask and you shall receive. Knock and it shall be opened to you." The answer might come a few days later in a flash of insight (usually when one is not even thinking about the question), in a dream, in a chance remark by somebody else, or in a book they happen to put into your hands. Here is a visualisation to help speed up the process:

"The Inner Healer" Visualisation

Lie down, and relax as deeply as you can, perhaps following the Alpha Plan described on pages 53–58. It is good to wear a blindfold for this visualisation, for you will be going deeper than in any visualisation you have done up until now and will need to cut out as much sensory stimulation from the outside as possible.

See yourself walking in beautiful natural surroundings. It could be anywhere that is meaningful to you, a forest perhaps,

*or along a river bank in the heart of the countryside. There
is nobody else around and you feel calm and peaceful.*

*Suddenly you hear somebody call your name from close by.
The voice is soft and so gentle that you are not afraid. You
pause to work out where the voice has come from. As if to
guide you, it repeats your name again and you move in that
direction. Soon you see who it is that called you. You feel a
strong sense of recognition, of having known this being all
your life. You feel very safe in its presence and intuit that it
loves you and wants the best for you.*

*The Being now speaks to you and says, "I am the Healer
Within. What do you need to know?" Ask a question, perhaps
"How can I heal myself of this illness?" and wait for the
reply. Whatever happens next is your answer, even if you may
not understand it immediately. Take it away with you and med-
itate on it. If it still didn't mean anything to you go back and
ask for clarification sometime later. Your Inner Healer is always available to you any time you need guidance for it is a
part of you, and the part of you that **Knows** how you are out
of balance, and what you need to restore that balance.*

Affirmations to Restore the Balance

I trust that I have the power to heal myself.
*I have learned the lesson(s) I needed to learn, and no longer
    need to be ill.*
*I have let go of any mental pattern that has been producing
    negative effects in my life.*
*My healing is complete on the plane of consciousness, and is
    now manifesting on the physical level.*
*I let go of all need for this illness, and allow it to disappear
    back into the nothingness from which it came.*

Seventh Chakra: Your Relationship to the Father, to Life, to the Whole.

The more seriously ill you know you are, the more your illness
comes to have, for want of a better word, a "religious" di-
mension. You will be forced to look at the possibility of death

and what this means to you. In making your will or other
arrangements, it may begin to dawn on you, possibly for the
first time at a feeling level, that you may not always be here.
It is always other people who die, never us, and death is the
biggest taboo in the Western World. We just don't talk about
it if we can possible help it. And yet, deep down, we know it
is the only certain thing, sooner or later, in everybody's future.

Whether or not your past life flashes before you in the best
tradition of penny dreadfuls, you will probably get to thinking
back over what you have experienced in your life and evalu-
ating these experiences by some sort of criteria which is meaningful to you. Perhaps too, for the first time, you might get to
thinking what it was all about—and in the process find yourself beginning to ask the "big" questions that are the domain
of religion. "What are we here for?" "Where did we come
from?" "What happens after death?" "Do we come back
again and again—or is that it?"

And whether or not it is God's Will that you be healed—
and ultimately He/She is the best judge of whether this is the
best thing for you at your present stage of evolution or whether
you have done what you needed to do this time round, and
He/She has other plans for you—it is good that you have the
leisure and the incentive to look at the deeper realities of Life.
In fact, avoiding doing so could have contributed to your illness, especially if you are middle-aged or elderly.

Jung's investigation of the archetypal layers of the Collec-
tive Unconscious led him to postulate the existence in all of
us of what he called a "religious function." It is expressed in
all cultures and in many different forms. In *Modern Man in
Search of a Soul* (see Further Reading) he pointed out that, in
our own culture, this religious function for very many people
has atrophied with the decline in the hold of organised religion
over their beliefs and values and the pinning of faith instead
in science, hedonism and materialism. Jung was struck by the
fact that the vast majority of patients in the second half of life
who came to him were ill or neurotic because their religious
function was not being expressed in some way in their lives.
In other words, they were living at too superficial a level, out
of touch with archetypal energies that, like a spring that dries
up, had disappeared underground. Their subjective experience

of this was that their lives lacked meaning (even though many of them were outwardly rich and successful), they felt dead inside, arid and sterile, "unreal."

Their way back to aliveness, renewal and wholeness was the unblocking of the Spring (itself, as at Lourdes, a potent symbol) and getting it to flow again often through working with the symbols that the patients produced in dreams. Jung remarked that often healing occurred if the person managed to find his or her way back into the religion they were brought up in but had later rejected.

The "non-religious" among us—possibly today a majority—no longer tend to relate to Life, the Universe, "It"—call it what you will—as a child to the parent which has given it birth and nurtures, protects and loves it (personalised in many religions as ("God the Father" or the "Great Mother"). Rather we look to science to conquer it, to render it safe, and, if we look at the escalating problem of pollution world-wide, in the process of the march of science, we are even raping our provider Mother Earth. And when it begins to dawn on us that in fact science is not infallible (for example, if our doctors cannot succeed with their pills and gadgets in making us well again) we may have very little in the way of inner resources to fall back on.

This is such a very personal and delicate area that I am afraid of rushing in where angels fear to tread. Working out my own relationship with It is an ongoing process. It is constantly surprising me. Whenever I think, "This is the way it is, what Life is all about," It comes at me from another angle as if to say "This also is part of the Whole—and this—and this." Life is mind blowing. It's bigger than us. We shall never "understand" it, just as the hand cannot grasp itself. The most we can do is to try to restore our feeling of connectedness with It, to get to realise that we are each a part of the Whole and a very special and valuable part. And if we can get to trust and surrender to It, then, however it seems on the outside, whether we get healed or not, whatever happens is good. Self-healing is like Life itself, paradoxical. We must put our total energy and commitment into doing whatever we need to do to bring it about—and be prepared to surrender with grace if that is what we are called to do.

Everything always works out, so it must be
working out NOW.
All is well, and all manner of things shall be well.
I trust that everything always happens as it should.
He's got the whole world in His hands—and that
includes ME.
I surrender to the Will of God.
Thy Will not mine be done.

part three

WELLNESS

*The great error in the treatment of the human
body is that physicians are ignorant of the
whole. For the part can never be well unless
the whole is well.*

—PLATO

fifteen

STAYING WELL

A state of wellness is something that those of us who are blessed with a strong constitution tend to take for granted, until it is no longer there. It is often only when one is confined to a sickbed, in pain perhaps or just feeling bad, or living in the shadow of some worrying and apparently insoluble problem that one really appreciates what a blessing it is to have a body that is functioning well and a mind at peace. Those who have managed to heal themselves after a bout of serious illness or breakdown will (hopefully) have learned not only not to take wellness for granted, but also the pathways to maintaining it.

What is "wellness?" We are used to defining illness—and indeed perhaps are better at labelling illnesses rather than curing them—but rarely find anyone attempting to define its opposite. And yet we know when we are experiencing wellbeing. We look good, we feel good, life feels worth living. Our bodies feel alive and full of energy, our state of mind is positive: yes, there may be problems to deal with, but we feel confident that we can do just that, our problems do not oppress or depress us. Emotionally we feel safe and that "God's in His Heaven and All's right with the world," a sort of optimism about the future and contentment with the way things are going. We feel good about ourselves and the people around us, and experience ourselves and them as lovable, or at least, not "out to get us." We are able to enjoy our work, to concentrate and be effective, and switch off, relax and play when the working day is over.

Martin Brofman suggests that if we can answer the following questions with a resounding "Yes," not only do our lives have quality, but we are safeguarded against the sort of stresses that can destroy our wellbeing. The questions to ask ourselves are:

1. Am I in the place I want to be?

2. Am I with the person I want to be with?

3. Am I doing what I want to do?

For Louise Hay, happiness is "feeling good about yourself." The experience (including my own) of those working in the caring professions—psychotherapists, healers, religious and social workers and, indeed, of medical men like Siegel and Simonton—as well as of those who have succeeded in healing themselves, suggests that a positive self-image and love for yourself is the essense of wellbeing. To feel that you *matter* and have something to offer, that your body is worth caring for, that you deserve a life of quality, that your relationships should reflect your innate lovability—these are not possible unless, deep down, you have a sense of self-worth, that you are as OK as anybody else.

Choosing to be kind to ourselves and to treat ourselves as well as we have been taught to treat others, is perhaps the most important choice we ever make in our lives, and it is an ongoing process, moment to moment. But it is only one of the choices we constantly have to make in order to safeguard our wellbeing. We are fortunate today in that we have more information to go on as to what is good for us and what isn't. We know all about the dangers, for example, of food additives, salmonella, cholesterol and salt; what is "junk food" and what isn't; about other health hazards like stress and pollution; more and more about what enhances and what wrecks our immune systems. Never before have so many people been so health-conscious, or had so many alternatives on offer for staying healthy: diets and food supplements, new forms of exercise, therapies, health clubs and farms and so forth. Each of us tends to swear by this or that, to give credit to, say, homoeopathic remedies or regular visits to the acupuncturist, or raw foods or macrobiotics, or the daily swim or jogging, for our continued wellbeing. Each of these things works for some people, and maybe not for others.

Perhaps the most important thing is not *what* we do, but the attitude implicit in the fact that we are doing it at all. As we have suggested earlier on, almost anything will work for you (including placebos) if you *believe* it will do you good. Perhaps the real therapeutic (and prophylactic) agent is our *intention* to enjoy wellbeing and to work for it, to consciously take charge of our own health. It is the total opposite to the victim consciousness which takes the attitude of "it must be something I ate" or "there's a lot of it around" that results in crowded GPs' surgeries night after night. And we have also seen how, in cases of catastrophic illness, the patients who decide to abandon their victim status and participate in their own healing process are the ones most likely to recover.

What is needed, therefore, for continued wellbeing is both a basic caring attitude towards ourselves and the commitment, arising naturally from that, to work with diligence to express it in our life-styles and the experiences we give ourselves. Our health is *our* responsibility, as is whether we experience quality in our lives or not. Of course we will make mistakes from time to time and end up feeling bad in some way or another. But every experience can be turned into a learning experience. And what we can learn when we go wrong—for example fatiguing ourselves by overdoing or over-commitment, suffering upset stomachs or hangovers through eating the wrong food and drinking the wrong drinks (or too much of them)—are our limits and the laws of cause and effect as they apply to us. For they are not the same for everybody. What you may be able to get away with in the way of late nights, for example, might reduce me to a near-zombie; the stress you get high on might be very draining for me; the crowd you like to hang out with I might find quite threatening and unable to relax with.

Each of us has different rhythms (including biorhythms), energy levels, nutritional, emotional and psychological needs, and they are constantly varying. Staying continually in touch with these as they change, and ensuring that our needs are met is essential, not only to feel good, but to stay well. And for this *self-awareness* is needed.

It would seem that when we lose this sense of self as an energy process and sensitivity to our needs—whether of our bodies or our psyches—that we are in for trouble and illness results. We have suggested that "dis-ease" manifests first as tension and subtle feelings of all not being well with us. If we are sufficiently aware of these early warnings, and not so busy and caught up with the world outside us that the line of communication between us and our innate "primitive" wisdom is down, these subtle energy imbalances and blockages can be remedied quickly, for example, by easing off the pressures upon us, by rest and relaxation, by giving attention to our diet, taking energy boosting supplements, using positive affirmations and visualisations, etc. Self-healing in this way is an ongoing process, to be applied whenever we feel out of sorts. It is the cultivation of an intimate relationship with one's own ongoing process, so that one always instinctively knows when one is overstepping one's limits—and what is needed to restore balance. Be more like an animal in this sense.

But it is impossible to cultivate this self-awareness if we do not give ourselves sufficient *space*. By "space" I mean psychological space: allowing yourself to withdraw for periods every day from "doing" into "feeling," from left-side brain activity into right-side brain *experiencing*, from functioning on the Beta brainwave frequency to relaxing into Alpha. How you arrange this is, as always, a question of preference. Some like to just put their feet up and relax, maybe listen to music; others will find it in restoring body awareness through exercise, jogging or swimming, perhaps; yet others in practising meditation or tai chi, or simply taking the dog for a walk in the park. It doesn't matter so long as what you get is the experience of having time for yourself, of not having to be "out there," relating, verbalising, meeting challenges, pressures and other people's time scales—and, in the process, usually cut off from in touchness with your body, your feelings and your emerging needs. Of course, most of us have to do this as part of earning a living. But it is essential to "come back in" to ourselves, to feel who we are again and what is going on with us, to listen to the messages that are all the time seeping up from the Unconscious about what is needed to stay whole, for inner balance.

One of the most healthful things we can do for ourselves is to make a point of structuring such a space into our daily routine for "switching off" and communing with ourselves, for sloughing off tension accumulated during the working day. Make it a priority, and be ruthless with outside demands for attention when it is your time to recharge your batteries. After all, if you get overstressed and fall ill, it will be your illness and not theirs. You owe it to yourself, and your loved ones as well. For it will be in these moments of quiet that you will be receptive to any subtle messages that perhaps all is not well in your body, or that you have some "unfinished business" that needs clearing—and can take appropriate action at this level when things are more easily handled.

Choosing to see things positively is also part of a commitment to feeling good and staying well. And how we see— whether it be ourselves, other people, situations, or Life generally—is always a choice, albeit sometimes a choice that we made long ago and have forgotten we ever did. Our wineglass can be either half-full or half-empty. Both are equally true, but which truth we choose carries a different experience with it, in this case, that of prosperity-consciousness or poverty-consciousness. We can choose to allow that person who is behaving so obnoxiously either to disturb, antagonise or threaten us, or we can expand our awareness to feel the place he or she is coming from (which is likely to be not a very uncomfortable place for them), and see them as somebody who perhaps has given up on love, is in pain, or otherwise is sending out messages in a maladaptive way.

This "expanding to include," whether what is included is a person, an idea, or one of our own feelings, is a kind of loving, an "allowing to be the way it is." Its opposite is resistance, judging, polarising against, or confrontation, all of which are demanding in terms of energy and often stressful or draining. It contracts us, which never feels good, and never does us (or the other) any good. Whenever you feel yourself tightening up ask yourself the question; "Is this really worth stressing myself for?''—and ''relax to include'' the potential stressor.

Commitment to staying well does not have to be a dreary business. Something that has long been suspected and has recently been validated by research is that doing things that make us feel good is beneficial to the immune system. Love, laughter and exercise we enjoy, relaxing, expressing ourselves freely, enjoying ourselves . . . here the pathways to wellbeing merge with the goal.

Pathways to Well-Being

1. Taking responsibility for your own health.

2. Commitment to caring for and nourishing yourself at all levels on a daily basis.

3. Becoming more sensitive to your changing energy levels and needs.

4. Taking space daily to relax and be with yourself.

5. Choosing to be positive.

6. Cutting out stress.

7. Accepting your feelings—*whatever* they are.

8. Being more playful and expressive—and finding things to enjoy.

9. Being more loving, forgiving, and accepting of others.

10. Learning more and more about who you are and what you need to be happy.

Human beings function as wholes. At any one time our living habits (what we are thinking, feeling, saying or doing) are either raising our vital energy and strengthening our resistance to disease, or depleting us. If we live in balance, contented and at peace with our environment and within ourselves, no germ has any power.

Let us now look at these pathways to wellbeing in more

detail, and see how we can apply them to nourishing ourselves at every level—body, mind, emotions and spirit.

CARING FOR OUR BODIES

Sound Nutrition

This is our first line of defence against illness.

GOOD	AVOID
vegetables	meat
vegetable oils	animal fats
raw foods	fried food
fish	processed foods
whole grains	adulterated foods
nuts, seeds	white flour products
fibre	sugar
fruit and fruit juices	alcohol
herb teas	coffee
garlic	salt

The following supplements should be taken at the first signs of energy depletion:

> Vitamins (especially C, high dose)
> Minerals (especially selenium and zinc)
> Ginseng (sparingly by women)

Exercise

We need to remind ourselves about how the body affects the mind as well as the other way round, the aspect that we have been giving more attention to throughout this book. Exercise is a great stress reliever: the sense of wellbeing we experience after it is probably due to the endorphins it releases into the bloodstream, which act rather like morphine. Exercise strengthens the heart and lungs, lowers blood pressure, increases the body's ability to dissolve clots, improves circulation and regulates the concentration of fats in the blood. A study in London among postal workers found that there was a lower incidence of heart attacks among those who delivered the mail than among those who had desk jobs. Exercise has also been found to be beneficial for asthma, especially swimming. In 1982, researchers established that those who do not exercise show more tension, fatigue, depression and anxiety than those who do.

That said, however, a word of caution. Exercising too strenuously, or too much too soon, can be harmful, if not positively dangerous, as the example of Jim Fixx shows. He took up running to help the heart disease from which he suffered, but did not change the high fat diet he had been on all his life—and died. Remember, too, that "exercise" need not be strenuous: stretching, yoga, dancing, and tai-chi are all forms of exercise too, and less dangerous than running yourself into the ground.

Adequate Sleep

Essential for keeping your energy levels up. You should know by now how many hours you need. Burning the midnight oil too often depletes energy levels and is just asking for trouble, especially if you have to work hard next day.

Regular Detoxification

Remember to drink three litres a day. Cleansing diets (e.g., brown rice or fruit juices or grapes, 2 lbs. a day) should be followed for a few days only, whenever you feel blown out, sluggish, or have been on a binge. Try also:

• Occasional fasting (one day only). It is essential to drink a lot while fasting.

• Massage, including self-massage (see pages 89–93).

• Saunas—sweat as much as you can and follow with a cold shower.

• Shower often—water is the biggest purifying agent there is. The reason one feels so fresh after taking a shower is not only to do with removal of sweat and grime. Water also cleanses your aura, your energy field that can be photogaphed using the Kirlian technique (and sometimes can actually be seen, if you are relaxed and look *past* another person).

You can also cleanse your aura as well by a form of self-massage that follows the lines of the acupuncture meridians. Here's how.

Aura Cleansing

1. Using the third and fourth fingers of both hands, press firmly on the point between the eyebrows. From there, with the same fingers, trace a line over the crown of the head down to the back of the neck and then down the spine as far as you can reach. Still using the same fingers, pick up at the point you left off and continue (pressing firmly down the centre of the back, the backs of the legs (simultaneously) to the calves. Finish with a flick of the fingers.

2. With the third and fourth fingers of the right hand start again at the point between the eyebrows and trace a line up and over the crown, down the back of the neck, along the left shoulder and the front of the left arm. Finish the movement with a sharp flick.

3. Repeat the above, this time using the third and fourth fingers of the left hand and tracing the line over the head and down the front of the right arm.

4. Using both hands, trace the line up from the point between the eyebrows over the head to the back of the neck. Here the hands separate, down each side of the neck under the jawline, over the front of the throat, to join up again at the breastbone. In one continuous flowing movement (and maintaining firm pressure) follow the centre line down the

front of the body with both hands, and then (simultaneously) down both legs, finishing at the ankles, once again with a flick.

Aura cleansing is good to do just before going to bed at night, and if you have been exposed to negative or scattered energy (for example, on a shopping spree in big, crowded stores, or travelling in the rush hour).

STAYING WELL WITH AIDS

It has been from America, with its longer exposure to AIDS, that the breakthroughs have mainly come, with well-documented cases of remissions and outright cures. Simon Martin's trail-blazing articles in *Here's Health* in the summer of 1987 entitled *I Didn't Know You Can Have AIDS and Get Better* brought to Britain news of some of these encouraging developments and how they were being achieved.

The physician and biochemist Russ Jaffe worked with 18 AIDS patients for 18 months. All achieved remission. Jaffe was interviewed by Michael Weiner on his approach. Jaffe had these recommendations to make (*Maximum Immunity*, see Further Reading):

1. Learn new patterns of consumption; this must be individualised. (By "new patterns of consumption" Jaffe explained that he meant new habits of thinking and relating—not least to oneself.)

2. Take balanced, non-irritating supplements.

3. Drink adequate amounts of "good for you" fluids (e.g., uncontaminated water, fruit juice, vegetable juice, fresh vegetable broth, soups, herb teas, etc.

4. Exercise appropriately for you.

5. Cultivate a relaxation reflex to reduce the cost of stress.

6. Breathe efficiently.

7. Commit yourself to expressing health in your life.

Persons with Aids in Europe are healing themselves too. Palle Johl, a young Dane diagnosed with AIDS in September 1987, got well again on the following régime that he adheres to strictly. Apart from one bout of flu, he remains symptom free:

> Vitamin C (10 gms daily, taken with lots of water)
> Beta-Carotene (25,000 IU daily)
> Vitamin E (55 IU daily)
> Selenium (200 mcg daily)
> Multivitamins and minerals
> Ipiroxo herb tea (strengthens immune system)
> Vegetarian diet to include a little fish: raw foods (carrots and beetroot especially good); beansprouts, nuts, humus, avocado, soymilk for protein; fruit—but don't eat at the same time as vegetables; vegetable oil
> No alcohol, drugs, tobacco, sugar, milk products, vinegar or yeast (to avoid candida)
> Exercise (don't overdo)
> Relaxation (including regular afternoon nap)
> Fresh air
> Meditation
> Visualisations
> Affirmations
> Chakra cleansing with sound and colour.

Palle also recommends sending the virus loving thoughts rather than negative ones, listening to one's own intuition, confronting the idea of one's own death and, very important, he told me, "Someone to talk to, either friends or a professional counsellor."

The "Staying Well with AIDS" Régime

This is a sound nutrition programme based on a mainly vegetarian diet:

- "Good for you drinks" (see page 174, especially daily fresh carrot and/or beetroot juice)

- Supplements (daily): high dose vitamin C: vitamin E; beta-carotene; acidophilus; vitamin B (whole complex); zinc; selenium (sparingly).

- Siberian ginseng; Evening Primrose Oil (see opposite).

- Detoxification: Caroline Myss advises strongly from her experience of healing AIDS patients that the following be totally cut out: alcohol, tobacco, recreational drugs, coffee, sugar.

- Exercise (non-competitive and non-strenuous).

- Deep relaxation sessions (daily).

- Positive, healing affirmations and visualisations, several times daily.

- Meditation (and/or prayer).

- Stress reduction (absolutely essential).

- Higher self-esteem (the most important single factor).

- Freer self-expression and finding things to enjoy.

- Complementary therapies (e.g., herbalism, acupuncture, homoeopathy) to stimulate the body's own healing power.

- Massage: for raising body energy (e.g., shiatsu), balancing or relaxation. One of the techniques taken from Reiki (a system of healing by touch) has been found to be effective in stimulating the thymus very quickly. Make fists, and with the knuckles tap rapidly up and down the breastbone, Tarzan-like. (Except that, instead of whooping like the Apeman, assist the process of stimulating your immune system as you rap away by thinking positive thoughts, e.g., visualising the thymus releasing T cells like a shower of sparks; saying a prayer; making an affirmation or simply thinking of somebody you love very much. A lot of PWAs are using this in California.

- Love and support; if necessary, ask for it—but get it.

As Jaffe suggested, the programme should be indivisualised to suit each patient, and what you have faith in will work for you. But sound nutrition, daily supplements, improved self-image and stress reduction are *essential* for repairing the immune system.

Evening Primrose Oil

Some alternative practitioners are using Evening Primrose Oil as part of an intensive nutritional programme with AIDS patients, and it is also being used at the Bristol Cancer Help Centre.

Evening Primrose is truly a remarkable plant, not least from the strange way it behaves. It has a curious habit of blooming, a few flowers at a time, only in the evening, and always at exactly the same time. In Denmark they have a lovely name for it, the "8 o'clock flower" (*klokken otte blomst*), though if you live in England you will have to allow for the one-hour time difference otherwise you will miss the phenomenon.

Since reading Judy Graham's book, *Evening Primrose Oil* (see Further Reading), on the therapeutic properties of the oil extracted from the flower I now regard the plant I have in my garden with something approaching awe.

The first disease for which Evening Primrose Oil was used was multiple sclerosis. It was found in 1974 to reduce the severity and frequency of relapses, and many people with MS have been taking it in capsule form ever since. Research carried out in the 1980s has shown its beneficial effect in the treatment of cancer in that it normalises tumours by stopping the cancer cells from multiplying, without affecting normal cells and without side effects. For this reason it is often given to patients at the Bristol Centre. In the case of AIDS, the oil, one of the most effective essential fatty acids, helps to keep cell membranes fluid and flexible and thus better able to cope with viral attack.

As more research is done, the list of ailments that respond favourably to Evening Primrose Oil lengthens. It is being used in the treatment of heart disease, vascular disorders and high blood pressure; diabetes; premenstrual syndrome; benign breast disease; rheumatoid arthritis; eczema and alcoholism. (Apparently the oil is good for avoiding hangovers too. Doctors researching its use in alcoholism found that taking four to six capsules before going to bed after drinking reduced appreciably the symptoms of a hangover.) Oil of Evening Primrose should always be taken with vitamin E, and ideally also with vitamin C, vitamin B6, nicotinamide (vitamin B3 or niacin), zinc and magnesium.

CONTROLLING OUR MINDS

We are not our minds. They are our computers. As with real computers, we should run the programmes we want, rather than be run by the computer. Our belief systems should support *us*, not the other way round. If an idea does not work for you, replace it with one that does. You may have to make a choice: do you want to be right, or do you want to be healthy and happy? Your mind can create heaven or hell, health or sickness for you. It makes a good servant, but the worst master in the world. Don't let it control you and bring you down. Tell it what to think.

REDUCE STRESS

Dr. Ray Rosenman, a Californian cardiologist and member of one of the leading heart research teams in the USA, believes that the biggest single reason why heart disease is the biggest single killer in the Western world today is the sheer pace of modern living. We are on the go all the time. Even when our bodies stop working, our minds are still at it, thinking, planning, worrying. We leak energy non-stop and then wonder why we feel drained and fatigued.

Together with his colleague Meyer Friedman, Rosenman conducted a now well-known investigation into which type of person was most likely to have a heart attack. Reminiscent of the cancer profiles we looked at in Part 1 they came up with a profile of the typical candidate for a coronary that they called Type A. They classified as Type A eighty San Franciscan men in business and the professions who were considered by people who knew them well to exhibit "a habitual sense of time urgency and excessive competitive drive." Rosenman and Friedman established a control group of men who did not show this sense of urgency or competitive drive and called them Type B. Type A was found to have had seven times more coronary heart disease than Type B, even though the diets and life-styles of the two groups were similar. Following this up, the researchers divided 3,500 healthy volunteers aged between 31 and 59 from Californian banks, businesses and airlines into Types A and B. They discovered ten years later that 250 of these volunteers had had heart attacks. Of these, 70 percent were Type As. None of the Type Bs had died.

You can check whether you are Type A by asking yourself the questions below, based on what their interviewers are trained to look for in the standard assessment interview. No cheating.

Are You Type A?

Do you:

- Bottle up your feelings?

- Speak emphatically?

- Often feel restless?

- Often frown, scowl, clench your teeth, clench your fist?

- Enjoy competition?

- Always play to win?

- Get irritated by being held up in traffic when driving?

- Frequently get upset or angry?

- Hate to be kept waiting, e.g., at a restaurant or in a bank?

- Prefer to do a job yourself rather than waiting for others to do it?

- Hate to leave jobs unfinished?

- Feel that time passes too quickly?

- Try to get work done while in the bathroom or eating alone?

- Try to get through jobs as quickly as you can?

- Like to walk fast?

- Look at your watch often during the day?

- Set yourself deadlines?

- Spend time on your hobbies only when you have nothing more important to do?

- Always turn up early for an appointment?

- Rarely stay at table long after dinner?

- Find yourself thinking of other things while talking to someone?

- Finish other people's sentences for them?

- Try to make others get to the point quicker?

Most people are a mixture of Type A and Type B. Rosenman and Friedman recognise four divisions in each group, from high risk (Type A1) to low risk (Type B4). If you answered "yes" to most of these questions, then you really must start slowing down and incorporating into your life-style periods of relaxation—and making them as much a priority as your work. Try to:

- Take frequent breaks and holidays.

- Lessen pressure of work (e.g., by rescheduling, delegating, extending deadlines, etc).

- Give yourself more time.

- Take more space for yourself to do what YOU want to do.

- Also you should use the daily Alpha Relaxation (see pages 53–58). "An Alpha a day keeps the doctor away." To antidote the damage caused by stress you have to learn to relax *deeply*, both mentally and emotionally as well as physically. "Just resting" is not enough. You might enrol for courses in one of the following to help you slow down: Transcendental Meditation; autogenic training; tai chi; or Silva Mind Control (the training devised by José Silva for developing the creative potential of the mind).

You should also try:

- Daily exercise (e.g., swimming).

- Cultivation of relaxing hobbies—preferably stimulating the right side of the brain and not involving much thinking (left-side brain activity).

- Enjoyment and laughter—the "best medicine." Remember, "The happy man (or woman) never gets cancer."

However you do it, you have to learn how to stop worrying and how to switch off your mind. This visualisation might help whenever you are in a panic about something, or worried about the outcome of a project and fretting over delays.

"Positive Outcome" Visualisation

Visualise something that you are anxious or worried about as being successfully completed. See yourself celebrating whatever it is. Who are you celebrating with and how? How does it feel to be able to relax again, knowing that everything is all right? Get this feeling firmly in your body—and remember it. Enjoy your fantasy for as long as you wish, feeling the tension of worry dissolving away. Later, after the visualisation is over, hold this feeling in your body of everything being OK—and recall it whenever you catch yourself starting to tighten up and worry.

Use this visualisation to give yourself confidence, help you relax, and programme yourself for success before embarking on some project that is important to you, e.g., going for a job interview, taking professional examinations, a business conference, or when you are steeling yourself for some personal encounter you are nervous about, e.g., with your bank manager.

Run a video in your head of everything going smoothly to perfection, just the way you would like it to go—and it i more likely to; you will be programmed for success.

Affirmations To Calm You Down

Cancel out with affirmations any negative things you tell your self in the course of the day. Here are a few you might use whenever you start to get tense, worried or uptight during the working day:

I have all the time in the world for what I want to do.
I release any thought that subjects me to any stress whatso ever.
It's OK to take my space whenever I need to.
I have my Workaholic firmly under control.
Easy is right.
I feel myself relaxing more and more.
Everything always works out, so it's working out NOW.
I trust that everything that happens is good.
This too shall pass.
There is no limit to how good I can feel.
Everything I touch is a success.
My work is a joy and a pleasure.
Money comes to me freely.
I can assert myself whenever I need to.
I now win at everything.
I love and approve of myself at all times.
Life is good—and gets better every day.
I feel totally safe at all times and with all people.
I forgive everybody I mistakenly thought ever hurt me.
I feel gratitude for my life and my many blessings.
I always get what I need.
My future is healthy, prosperous, exciting and totally SAFE.
My life is full of love, joy, success and prosperity.
People give to me freely: I do not have to beg or fight.
Strangers are friends to me.
I am special, magnificent and deserving only of the best.
All I have to do is to relax, trust and enjoy.

sixteen

ACCEPTING AND EXPRESSING OUR FEELINGS

Whenever we lie about our true feelings to ourselves or to others we depress our immune systems a little more. Risk saying "NO" whenever you are clear you don't want to do something. If you are not clear, ask for more time. To "string along" when everything inside you is shouting "NO" is bad enough: you won't enjoy it, that's for sure. And then to pretend you did to be polite merely compounds the outrage to your integrity.

Accept your feelings *whatever* they are. There is always a reason for them. Instead of judging and repressing them, rather try to understand them and how they are trying to protect you. For example:

Anger

The feeling we are all afraid of, in ourselves and others. Never suppress anger. Its biological function is to protect you—your space, sense of worth, your possessions—perhaps some day, even your life. Without the capacity to feel anger you are defenceless and a pushover. If you suppress it the adrenalin will poison your body and depress your immune system. Risk confronting the person you are angry with. Don't blame or play victim. Just tell them directly you feel angry and why.

Don't waste your energy telling them how *THEY* should be. Stick with telling them in detail how *YOU* feel. Perhaps they'll get to understand something about themselves, e.g., how insensitive they can be, perhaps not. But *you* will feel a whole lot better.

If for some reason it is inappropriate, impossible or too risky to express your anger directly, tell yourself you will deal with your anger as soon as you can. And when you can, put out the anger energy physically in some way. Use your whole body and let sounds come.

For example you could:

• Strangle a cushion. Really murder it!

• Wring the neck of a towel.

• Retire to your room and throw a tantrum. You've probably never dared to do this since you were little and couldn't get your own way, so let me remind you of the art of tantrum-throwing. First and foremost, to be a good tantrum it has to be total, using the whole body and putting all your energy into it. Take your shoes off, lie on your back on your bed. Make fists and start to bring them down on the mattress, not together but alternately, left fist, right fist and so on. When you get a rhythm, keep on doing it, harder and harder, and at the same time start kicking into the mattress with your heels, once again alternately. At first you may not be in touch with being angry anymore. But if you persevere with punching and kicking, you will. And when you do, let it all hang out. Go wild and beat the mattress as fast and hard as you can.

• Dance your anger away. Put on some heavy rock music, preferably fast and loud, and dance as furiously and energetically as you can until you start to enjoy the dancing for its own sake.

• Go for a run in the park.

• Go for a swim—and put all your energy into swimming length after length until you feel tired.

One of the outlets I used to allow myself (and when I have told friends this they have said with some relief, ''Oh, do you do that as well?'') was to sit in the car with the windows closed and just scream, shout and swear. It doesn't have to make sense. Just let all the rubbish out the way it wants to come. It's only raw energy, and it's better out than in. Never visualise hurting anyone or harm coming to them.

And don't dump your anger on anyone who comes within range. They don't deserve it—and you'll only get it back or feel guilty later.

Guilt

According to Gestalt therapy, guilt is resentment turned inwards against the self. It is the most useless and one of the most damaging feelings we can harbour. So, if you are beating yourself up with guilt, ask yourself the questions ''Who would I like to beat up if it were possible?'' and ''Why am I angry with that person?'' In most cases you will find that you are subconsciously angry because in some way you have allowed that person to trap you into their reality, to manipulate you into meeting their expectations, perhaps to take responsibility for them.

Take back your power. The only person you are responsible for is yourself. And by colluding with somebody playing helpless you are not helping them to realise their own power, but confirming their self-imposed status of victim. Rather, encourage them to take responsibility for themselves and realise the choice they have made and the choices that are open to them. And never, NEVER put yourself down and never let anyone make you feel guilty for being who you are and exercising your birthright to live how you want to live. Don't make their self-limiting ideas yours. A lifeline when you are feeling really guilty is the ''Gestalt Prayer'':

You are you and I am me.
I am not in this world to meet your expectations.
You are not in this world to meet mine.
I am here to do my thing.
You are here to do your thing.

Sometimes we will meet—and that's beautiful.
Sometimes we won't. Too bad.

Jealousy

Another heavy feeling, and one that we judge harshly. Really, there is no such thing as "jealousy." If you give yourself the space to look into what you are really experiencing instead of avoiding feeling the unpleasant turmoil within by either acting out or denying, you will find anger, fear, vulnerability, hurt . . . For most of us it is easier to get angry than to admit to feeling hurt, vulnerable or afraid.

Acknowledge your own anger—but also acknowledge the other person's freedom to do what they need to do for themselves. Blaming never does any good: all it provokes is resistance and counter-attack. Sharing your hurt, vulnerability and fear without trying to manipulate or blame is non-threatening to the other person and more likely to bring back lost love, holding or at least real communication—which is really what your Inner Child needs.

Fear

The way not to let yourself be controlled and manipulated by fear is to confront it head-on. As with all emotions, allowing yourself to experience them totally makes them disappear. If you resist them, think you shouldn't feel this way, blame yourself for feeling whatever it is—you're stuck with them. The nature of energy is to move, to change into something else, and feelings are energy. It is impossible to go on feeling the same for very long unless you yourself are hanging on to a feeling and continually re-creating it.

Get to know your fear. How does it feel to be afraid? Where in your body does fear "live"? What, specifically, are you afraid of? What is the worst that could happen? So what? If you keep on asking yourself "So what"? you get to realise that your catastrophic expectations are maybe not really taken so seriously after all. When you really look into fear it evaporates, just as darkness clears when light is brought. For, like darkness, fear is not an entity in itself, but the absence of love. And, ultimately, all fear is the fear of loss of love by the Inner Child, to whom it feels like death.

Vulnerability

Allowing yourself to be vulnerable is not weakness but a sign of strength. Intimacy is impossible without it. Trying to be invulnerable may stop you from getting hurt. But it also stops any goodies from reaching you. And if you can allow yourself to show your vulnerability the chances are the person or persons you are with will feel they too have permission to do likewise. Which makes for a nice, soft, heart-centred vibration between you.

Of course, it goes without saying that you have to be aware enough of whether it is safe for you in any given situation to allow your vulnerability to show. But always acknowledge it to yourself, whether or not you choose to share it. Be gentle and understanding with your vulnerability, for it is your Inner Child asking for your support. Appreciate it, for without it you would not be able to *feel*. And the recovery of our capacity to feel, to experience the life force within us, is very much a part of the healing process.

Giving and Receiving Love

Love:

• Heals us.

• Heals others.

• Strengthens immunity.

• Energises.

• Is quality of life.

• Antidotes fear.

• Dispels nightmares.

• Relieves pain.

• Is the opposite of judgement.

• Respects our own and others' freedom.

• Sweetens relating.

• Is the only thing big enough to transcend and include opposites.

• Is a willingness to share another's reality, even if we don't understand it.

• Makes us willing to listen rather than trying to convince.

• Accepts difference instead of trying to kill it.

• Transforms negative into positive energy.

Love truly "makes the world go round." Our only real protection against the uncertainties and unpredictability of life is our capacity to love and receive love. It is the only thing that makes us feel really safe, held. Everything else is merely taking out insurance. Without love we feel like aliens on this planet. We have seen how the biggest single factor in keeping us alive and well is loving and feeling loved. Without it, not only do we not grow and flourish, we dry up and wither, just as surely as do our thymuses.

At the opposite pole to love are indifference, judging, excluding, intolerance, harbouring grudges and refusing to forgive. These mental attitudes are dangerous for our health. There is a cold, hard, biting, acid quality of energy about them that bodes ill for the soft, warm tissues of the body on to which they unleash their chemical messengers.

Love relaxes us, and that goes beyond the euphoria that follows love-making. With trust and the achievement of intimacy, paranoia dissolves, and with it the need to keep our defences up—which means an immune system constantly on red alert. Not only is our own energy conserved, but we become energised by opening ourselves to the loving vibrations of others.

Love heals. And that means, as we have seen, "making whole." It is the royal path to "at-one-ment" through the cultivation of good will and understanding. On the individual level love is necessary for the integration of body, mind and spirit; in relationships between people it is vital for harmonious and cooperative sharing of the planet that is our joint home; and in our relationship to life, trusting that "All is well, and all manner of things shall be well"—however it looks in our darkest hours.

And loving, like everything else, is a *choice*. At every moment, in every encounter with another, or in every thought about ourselves, we have a choice: either to judge or to try to understand; to contract and reject or expand to include; to resist and polarise against this particular manifestation of energy or to allow it to be, just the way it is. And the miracle is, as proved time and time again, for example in psychotherapeutic practice, that it is through acceptance and understanding that transformation happens.

You don't have to like something in order to love it. *Flow, don't fight.* Just to be willing to respect its right to exist is enough. It has been found, for example, that visualisations of viruses or cancer cells being destroyed violently tend to make the patient worse rather than better. A more gentle, respectful approach is more effective, which could include entering into dialogue with them to find out what message they bring and learning from them about why they are there and what changes you need to make in your life.

Love as much as you can and in any way you know how, starting with yourself. And not only other human beings but the animal and plant kingdoms as well. It is the best thing you can do, not only to stay well, but to help heal our Mother the Earth, who is in pain right now as a result of our lack of respect and care for her.

As well as putting out as much love as you can, allow yourself to receive it. It's free. And you deserve it, simply for being who you are. Which is lovable, magnificent, and special.

FURTHER READING

The following is a short list of useful books that are all very readable:

Michael Blate: *How to Heal Yourself Using Foot Acupressure* (Falkynor Books)

———. *How to Heal Yourself Using Hand Acupressure* (Falkynor Books)

Penny Brohn: *Gentle Giants* (David & Charles)

———. *The Bristol Programme* (David & Charles)

Norman Cousins: *Anatomy of an Illness* (Norton)

John Davidson: *Subtle Energy* (The C. W. Daniel Co.)

Shakti Gawain: *Creative Visualization* (Bantam)

———. *Living in the Light* (New World Library)

Louise Hay: *You Can Heal Your Life* (Hay House)

———. *You (Can Heal Your Body* (Hay House)

Brian Ingles and Ruth West: *The Alternative Health Guide* (Knopf)

Leslie Kenton: *Raw Energy Recipes* (Arrow)

Leslie and Susannah Kenton: *Raw Energy* (Warner Books)

Louis Proto: *Coming Alive* (Sterling)

————. *Take Charge of Your Life* (Sterling)

————. *Who's Pulling Your Strings?* (Sterling)

————. *Total Relaxation in Five Steps: The Alpha Plan* (Penguin)

————. *Meditation for Everybody* (Penguin)

Sadhya Rippon: *The Bristol Recipe Book* (Random Century)

Meir Schneider: *Self Healing: My Life and Vision* (Arkana)

Jason Serinus: *Psychoimmunity and the Healing Process* (Celestial Arts)

C. Norman Shealy and Carolyn Myss: *AIDS: Passageway to Transformation* (Stillpoint)

————. *Transformation* (Stillpoint)

————. *Breaking Through Illness* (Stillpoint)

————. *The Creation of Health* (Stillpoint)

Bernie Siegel: *Love, Medicine and Miracles* (HarperCollins)

Carl and Stephanie Simonton: *Getting Well Again* (Bantam)

Dr. Rosy Thomson: *Loving Medicine* (Gateways)

Michael Weiner: *Maximum Immunity* (Pocket Books)

RESOURCES

Tapes for Healing, Relaxation, Meditation

Creative Audio
8751 Osborne, Dept. B
Highland, IN 46322
(tapes of relaxation and guided visualization)

Effective Learning Systems, Inc.
Dept. A
5221 Edina End Blvd.
Edina, MN 55435
(tapes of relaxation and guided visualization)

Halpern Sounds
1775 Old Country Road, Apt. 9
Belmont, CA 94002
(tapes of new age music by Steve Halpern)

Louise Hay: *Morning and Evening Meditations*
———. *Cancer: Your Healing Power*
———. *AIDS: A Positive Approach*

————. *Self-Healing*
————. *What I Believe/Deep Relaxation*

Obtainable from:
Hay House
P.O. Box 2212
Santa Monica, CA 90407/2212

Carolyn Myss: *The Challenge of AIDS*
(package containing 70-page booklet and 3 healing tapes)
Obtainable from:
Stillpoint Publishing, Dept. G
P.O. Box 640
Walpole, NH 03608

Source Cassettes
Dept. M176
P.O. Box W
Stanford, CA 95305
(tapes of affirmation and visualization by
Emmett E. Miller, M.D.)

Tools for Change
Dept. P, P.O. Box 14141
San Francisco, CA 94114
(tapes on applied meditation)

Therapies

American Association of Acupuncture & Oriental Medicine
1424 16th Street N.W. Suite 105
Washington, DC 20036
Tel: 1-202-265-2287
(referrals to local practitioners)

American Botanical Council
P.O. Box 201660
Austin, TX 78720
Tel: 1-512-331-8868

American Herb Association
P.O. Box 99
Rescue, CA 95672

Aphrodisia
282 Bleecker Street
New York, NY 10014
Tel: 1-212-989-6440
(for mail order catalog send $2.00)

Ayurvedic Medicine
Maharishi Ayurveda Association of America
P.O. Box 282
Fairfield, IA 52556
Tel: 1-515-472-8477

British Association for Autogenic Training
101 Harley Street
London W1
England

The Cancer Support and Educational Center
250 Oak Grove Avenue
Menlo Park, CA 94025

Center for Attitudinal Healing (founded by Gerald G. Jampolsky, author of *Love is Letting Go of Fear*.
21 Main Street
Tiburon, CA 94920
Tel: 1-415-435-5022

Dr. Edward Bach Healing Society
644 Merrick Road
Lynbrook, NY 11563
(for Bach flower remedies)

Ellon, (Bach USA) Inc.
P.O. Box 320
Woodmere, NY 11598
(for Bach flower remedies)

Flower Essence Services
P.O. Box 586J
Nevada City, CA 05959
(for Bach flower remedies)

Herb Research Foundation
1007 Pearl Street Suite 200
Boulder, CO 80302
Tel: 1-303-449-2265
(for information on herbs)

Russell M. Jaffe, M.D., Ph.D.
2177 Chaisn Bridge Road
Vienna, VA 22180
Tel: 1-703-255-9834

Elisabeth Kübler-Ross
Shanti Nilaya
South Point 616
Head Waters, VA 24442
Tel: 1-703-396-3441
(for newsletter and list of mail order books, tapes and videos)

The Native Herb Company
Box 742 S
Capitola, CA 95010
(information on herbs)

The National Center for Homeopathy
801 N. Fairfax Street Suite 306
Alexandria, VA 22314
Tel: 1-703-548-7790
(for information about homeopathic practitioners)

The Nevada Clinic
3720 Howard Hughes Parkway
Las Vegas, NV 89109
(holistic health clinic, using homeopathic and other treatments)

Pegasus Products
P.O. Box 228
Boulder, CO 80306
(for flower essence therapy)

The San Francisco Healing Project
513 Valencia Street
San Francisco, CA 94110
Tel: 1-415-558-9292
(telephone referral service for alternative and holistic practitioners and resources)

The Simonton Center
Dept. W, P.O. Box 1055
Azle, TX 76020
(tapes, books and details of the 5-day New Patient Session program)

Hal Stone, M.D.
Thera, P.O. Box 604
Albion, CA 95410-0604
Tel: 1-707-937-4329
(for details of sessions and courses in Voice Dialogue, a useful tool for uncovering subconscious programs and motivations with regard to illness and resistance to getting well again, developed by Dr. Stone and Dr. Sidra Winkelman.)

T. H. Enterprises
1200 N. Lake Avenue
Pasadena, CA 91104
(Touch for Health—applied kinesiology)

Zephyrus
(The London Center for Voice Dialogue)
3 Trevor Street
London SW7 1DU
England

(For more awareness of who you are and your hidden motives
for doing what you do. Not a therapy but a fascinating way
to understand the different parts of you and how they influence
you.)

INDEX